Hospital-Based Integrative Medicine

A Case Study of the Barriers and Factors Facilitating the Creation of a Center

Ian D. Coulter • Marcia A. Ellison • Lara Hilton
Hilary J. Rhodes • Gery Ryan

T0146314

Supported by the National Center for Complementary
and Alternative Medicine

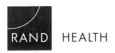

RAND HEALTH

This work was supported by the National Center for Complementary and Alternative Medicine. The research was conducted in RAND Health, a division of the RAND Corporation.

Library of Congress Cataloging-in-Publication Data

Hospital-based integrative medicine : a case study of the barriers and factors facilitating
    the creation of a center / Ian D. Coulter ... [et al.].
        p. cm.
    Includes bibliographical references.
    ISBN 978-0-8330-4559-1 (pbk. : alk. paper)
    1. Integrative medicine. 2. Hospitals—United States—Planning—Case studies.
I. Coulter, Ian D., 1945– II. Rand Corporation.
    [DNLM: 1. Hospital Administration—United States. 2. Complementary
Therapies—United States. 3. Delivery of Health Care, Integrated—United States.
4. Hospital Planning—United States. 5. Organizational Case Studies—United
States. WX 150 H8233 2008]

R733.H676 2008
362.11068—dc22

                                                                2008034971

The RAND Corporation is a nonprofit research organization providing objective analysis and effective solutions that address the challenges facing the public and private sectors around the world. RAND's publications do not necessarily reflect the opinions of its research clients and sponsors.

RAND® is a registered trademark.

Cover photo courtesy of the Samueli Institute

Published 2008 by the RAND Corporation
1776 Main Street, P.O. Box 2138, Santa Monica, CA 90407-2138
1200 South Hayes Street, Arlington, VA 22202-5050
4570 Fifth Avenue, Suite 600, Pittsburgh, PA 15213-2665
RAND URL: http://www.rand.org/
To order RAND documents or to obtain additional information, contact
Distribution Services: Telephone: (310) 451-7002;
Fax: (310) 451-6915; Email: order@rand.org

Preface

This report presents the results of a five-year study of a hospital-based center for integrative medicine (IM). The objective was to identify the barriers to and facilitators of developing and implementing IM programs.

The study used a longitudinal case study method to track the establishment of a single hospital-based IM center. Using extensive qualitative interviews, the project staff conducted a stakeholder analysis of all participants involved in the establishment and operation of the center. The respondent sample included board of directors members, hospital administrators, medical staff, integrative medicine providers, attending physicians, community physicians, community-based providers of complementary and alternative medicine (CAM), and patients who visited the IM center. In addition to interviews, data were collected from hospital documents, patient files, patient questionnaires, and provider questionnaires.

During the study, the IM center was dismantled as an independent clinic. This report, therefore, tells a story of both creation and demise.

The findings should be of interest to those involved in IM centers, those who are contemplating creating such centers, and those who are interested in researching such centers.

This work was supported by the National Center for Complementary and Alternative Medicine. This work was conducted in RAND Health, a division of the RAND Corporation. A profile of RAND

Health, abstracts of its publications, and ordering information can be found at http://www.rand.org/health/.

Contents

Figures

Tables

Summary

No uniform definition of integrative medicine (IM) exists, but current IM practices in hospital settings involve some form of partnership between complementary and alternative medicine (CAM) and biomedicine. Given the historic and very public animosity between CAM and biomedicine, integrating them might seem a daunting task.

Despite this challenge, a growing number of attempts have been made to incorporate CAM into the institutional home of biomedicine, the hospital. While the literature is full of anecdotal reporting on some of these attempts, no rigorous, in-depth analysis has been conducted that isolates the factors that facilitate integration and those that act as barriers.

This study arose out of a request for applications (RFA) from the National Center for Complementary and Alternative Medicine for research "to identify barriers and facilitators to the integration of CAM and conventional health care practices."

The study adopted a longitudinal methodology to track the establishment of a single hospital-based IM center. As it turned out, this was also a study of the unexpected collapse of the center. Thus, the report tells the story of the center's creation and demise.

Using extensive qualitative interview data, the project staff conducted a stakeholder analysis of all participants involved in the establishment and operation of the center. The respondent sample included members of the board of directors, hospital administrators, medical staff; IM providers, attending physicians; community physicians, community-based CAM providers, and patients. In addition to interviews, data were collected from hospital documents, patient files, patient questionnaires, and provider questionnaires.

The analysis follows the story of the center, which has three parts: planning, implementation, and demise. Each part was characterized by internal and external factors that both helped and hindered the establishment and operation of the center.

This case study represents what might be termed the first generation of integrative medicine. With few models and no experience in creating such a clinic, the hospital made some decisions in the areas of administration, finance, and legal issues that created barriers. The business model was based on faulty assumptions and projections; it did not adequately anticipate or address the challenges of practicing CAM in the hospital setting. The legal structure created to protect the center and the hospital (a professional corporation) proved to be a major barrier to the center's success as an economic enterprise. On the other hand, factors that many thought would harm the center, such as medical opposition, turned out to be less of a problem than expected.

Some factors clearly worked in favor of the IM center, including a perception of strong support from the board of directors. Both the board and the Medical Executive Committee approved the plan to implement a research-based CAM program, and the fact that the IM center was initiated by the chief of medicine had a significant impact. The reputation of the hospital contributed to the success of the project—the institution is known for initiating innovative programs and meeting community needs.

There was evidence (albeit misinterpreted) of a large consumer demand for CAM, and it appeared to be a clear, untapped revenue source. An organizational home was found for the new IM center in the hospital foundation. Set up as a consultative practice, it did not pose an economic threat to other hospital programs.

The fact that the key players in the center were western-trained biomedical doctors (internal medicine) also helped allay fears about "voodoo medicine." The implementation of a hospital-wide credentialing procedure that included hospital privileges was a major accomplishment that allowed the appointment of CAM providers.

However, more factors militated against than for the success of the center. It was established during an economic downturn in the health field. The business plan included unrealistic expectations and financial projections, and there was no strategic plan, vision, operating budget, or marketing research. The professional corporation created for the center turned out to be an enormous barrier to its success.

The center's location, design, and décor also held it back. It never became an integral part of the hospital. Its space was inadequate and not "prestigious," and it was located in an area where many competitors provided CAM services.

The center was obliged to take the insurance provided for hospital employees, as well as Medicare and Medi-Cal, which had a drastic impact on its ability to generate a profit. Supplements and herbs were sold by the hospital pharmacy rather than by the center.

Widespread skepticism about the center hindered broad-based referral of patients within the hospital, and many departments already had their own CAM therapies in place.

Ironically, the institution's prestigious reputation made the medical staff wary about bringing in CAM modalities. Many felt that the center was a threat to their credibility.

The corporate structure that gave the center regulatory freedom and independence from oversight also made it impossible to shift costs or bury any losses, and the time frame allotted for its success was insufficient.

As a proposed center for research, it lacked the infrastructure necessary to conduct research. Further, the clinical and education demands were high, leaving little time for research.

Many of the CAM providers the center wanted to hire lacked appropriate licensure and were not familiar with hospital protocols and the referral process.

In terms of survival, the center ultimately was not successful. But if it is judged in terms of its achievements, it can be called successful.

In retrospect, the center was expected to do too much, too fast. In fact, it was surprising that the creators and participants achieved the results they did. They managed to take a vision, create a center in a highly bureaucratic and somewhat skeptical environment, hire CAM providers, open for business, develop a clientele, and provide services with which clients, for the most part, were satisfied. The center and its outreach efforts promoted the integration of CAM and biomedicine, and various CAM modalities are still being practiced in this institution today.

Ultimately, however, the IM center's impact may become apparent only in years to come. By thinking outside the box, the creators of this program dared to merge CAM and biomedicine under the same roof. Their example has already inspired two staff members to establish IM centers elsewhere and will likely inspire more attempts.

The most apt metaphor for our findings about the center might be that of evolution. At the end of the process, some forms of CAM and IM survived within the hospital. These were the modalities that adapted. The IM center itself, as it was initially conceived, did not adapt and did not survive. For those contemplating creating a center of integrative medicine in a hospital setting, the story suggests some facilitators of and barriers to survival that merit close scrutiny.

Acknowledgments

This project was funded by a grant from the National Center for Complementary and Alternative Medicine (NCCAM) (Grant No. R01AT00872). The authors of the report are responsible for its content. Statements in the report should not be construed as endorsement by NCCAM or the U.S. Department of Health and Human Services.

The authors wish to thank those who agreed to be interviewed as part of this study; the report would not have been possible without them.

We also wish to thank Leigh Rohr for her contribution to the preparation of the report; Louise Parker for her contributions to research design and data collection; and Harlinah Lopez for her data collection efforts.

We also wish to acknowledge the contribution of Dr. Mary Hardy, who played a key role in the initiation of this study and its implementation.

CHAPTER ONE

Introduction

The overall goal of this in-depth case study was to document the barriers to and facilitators of integrating biomedicine and complementary and alternative medicine (CAM) in a hospital-based integrative medicine (IM) center. The process of establishing an IM center in a hospital brought to the forefront long-standing tensions and changing attitudes of biomedical and CAM practitioners, and highlighted the factors that impede or facilitate integration. An IM center represents two distinct medical systems and philosophies. Biomedicine, with its disease focus and fairly homogeneous, vertically organized hierarchy of specialists and generalists, traces its philosophical roots and practices to rationalistic, quantitative western scientific traditions. In contrast, CAM is a loosely organized aggregation of heterogeneous practices based on global medical systems and philosophies that approach health and illness from an individualized but holistic perspective (Coulter, 2004; Kaptchuk and Miller, 2005). Moreover, while biomedical managed care practices seek to limit the time physicians spend with each patient, CAM typically depends on extensive intake processes and lengthy or repeated individualized treatments. Given these significant differences and the long-standing antipathy between biomedicine and CAM, some argue that any attempt to integrate these strikingly different medical paradigms detracts from both and results in greater risks and dubious benefits for practitioners and patients alike (Kaptchuk and Miller, 2005). Despite these concerns, integration has been occurring in some form for over a decade (Dalen, 1998; Barrett, 2003; Cohen, 2004; Coulter and Willis, 2004; Jonas, 2005; Ruggie, 2005; Eisenberg, 2006). This case study examines an attempt to institutionalize the process by establishing a hospital-based IM center.

Definition of Integrative Medicine

An immediate difficulty in understanding this area is that no uniform definition exists for CAM (Coulter and Willis, 2004), let alone a consensus about what constitutes integration. The National Center for Complementary and Alternative Medicine (NCCAM) in the United States defines CAM as "healthcare practices that are not an integral part of conventional medicine. As diverse and abundant as the peoples of the world, these practices may be grouped within five major domains: alternative medical systems; mind-body interventions; biologically based treatments; manipulative and body-based methods; and energy therapies" (NCCAM, 2001–2005). The University of Arizona's Program in Integrative Medicine defines integrative medicine as "healing-oriented medicine that takes account of the whole person (body, mind, and spirit), including all aspects of lifestyle. It emphasizes the therapeutic relationship and makes use of all appropriate therapies, both conventional and alternative" (University of Arizona).

However, as CAM is increasingly sought by patients and included in teaching programs in medical schools and in medical practice, the distinction between CAM and biomedicine is problematic. Concomitantly, there is increasing difficulty naming the alternative to CAM; it is variously called *mainstream medicine, conventional medicine, orthodox medicine, allopathic medicine, modern western medicine, scientific medicine, and biomedicine.* As noted in Wiseman (2004), each of these labels presents difficulties, because none of them clearly distinguish this form of medicine from much of CAM. We concur with Wiseman, who suggests that the term biomedicine is the least evaluative of the labels and denotes a medicine within which the biological sciences are a core component and where explanations for disease and illness are predominantly biologically based (Mead and Bower, 2000). Further, the diversity of practices included under the rubric of CAM lessens its usefulness as an umbrella term. These practices range from very focused therapies such as reflexology to whole medical systems such as Ayurvedic medicine and traditional Chinese medicine.

The issue of what to call the CAM modalities has important social and political ramifications. To call these heterogeneous modalities *alternative* may be to claim too much for their role in health care, but to call them *complementary* may make their role seem secondary to primary medical care. To call them *integrative* implies some process in which integration or convergence occurs, which may or may not be true. And even if it does occur, the term does not capture the nature of the integration or the process by which it has been achieved. The current label, *individualized medicine* (Hyman, 2005), may alleviate as well as obfuscate the benefits, risks, and issues inherent to integration.

Many supporters of integrative medicine recognize three approaches to integration with biomedicine: incorporate (1) CAM therapies that have passed rigorous scrutiny; (2) those that have passed the test of time; or (3) those that are credentialed or licensed. But CAM is more than simply a set of therapeutic interventions. These interventions are given in the context of a distinct health encounter and often within a distinct philosophy of health and health care, both of which may influence the effectiveness of the intervention (Coulter, 1999). There have also been increasing attempts to incorporate CAM in existing biomedical institutions. In the United States, institutional integrative medicine is being developed in a highly individualistic manner, and the body of literature documenting attempts to establish integrative centers is growing (Moore 1997; Blanchet, 1998; Muscat, 2000; Weeks, 2001; Barrett, 2003). The co-occurring increase in the widespread use of CAM by the public and the attempts to institutionalize this use in biomedical clinics imply a major social/cultural shift.

At the most fundamental level, an IM clinic brings together those who offer a service (biomedical providers) and those who offer what can be perceived as an adjunctive or competitive service (IM/CAM providers); those who regulate integration (administrators); and those who seek a service (IM/CAM patients). Each group has a distinct stake in integrative medicine, and they may be in conflict. Moreover, integrating an IM center into a hospital setting requires a change not only in the attitudes of medical staff but in the relationship between CAM providers and the hospital as well. Patients also must accept the use of CAM. From a social and cultural perspective, for CAM to be fully integrated, it must become a seamless part of a social nexus uniting these numerous stakeholders.

Institutional Integration

In 2003, a national survey of 1,007 U.S. hospitals documented that 16 percent provided IM and over one-quarter (26.7%) offered some form of CAM (Larson, 2005). Patient demand was the most significant factor (83%) for incorporating IM/CAM. Novey (in Larson, 2005) suggests that the models of integration that have been implemented can be divided into five types. The most prevalent type, the "virtual" model, characterizes 75 percent of hospital-based programs. This model is also known as the "clinic without walls," as CAM services are dispersed throughout a hospital or medical system. It requires little internal restructuring and adds little additional cost, as it typically uses existing medical staff to add complementary services (e.g., physical therapists provide therapeutic massage). In contrast, consultatory models, either general or focused on a particular medical specialty, rely on referrals from staff physicians to in-house CAM providers, with the referring physician maintaining responsibility for the patient. The third model—primary care that integrates CAM and biomedicine—is the least common according to Novey, because it positions IM/CAM providers in direct competition with staff physicians. The fourth model—fitness or wellness centers—may provide a funnel system for accessing CAM providers. Likewise the increasingly popular fifth model, which (while more closely aligned with the hotel and service industries) caters to high-end clients who are willing to pay out of pocket for expensive CAM services in a retreat-like environment.

Novey outlines eight elements of successful integration. The first, *adequate marketing research*, ensures that the model fits community and staff interests as well as a local niche market. The second element, a *viable business plan*, stresses the need for realistic projected revenues, controlling overhead costs, securing at least three to five years of administrative commitment as well as support from key internal administrative executives, and including "anchor" services (i.e., those that are reimbursable) to secure a broad payer mix. The services that can provide economic anchors will vary by state-specific third-party reimbursement policies. The third core element of successful integration is *anticipating "bear traps,"* such as unrealistic expectations from administrative executives or fears of competition from biomedical staff, and avoiding these pitfalls through sustained networking and education. The fourth element is to *secure a solid referral base*, establishing a pattern of reciprocal referrals and appropriate follow-up. The fifth element, *hiring appropriate staff*, entails more than just establishing their credentials and training, and running criminal background checks. In addition, Novey suggests, candidates should demonstrate their skills by providing treatment to a staff member. The sixth element is *building a CAM/IM team through regular meetings*, which may be particularly important for CAM providers who are accustomed to practicing independently. Novey recognizes *front office staff* as the seventh element of success, as they provide a safety net for those wary of CAM by recognizing and mitigating the "pathway of risk" from their first contact to ensuring accurate and timely follow-up practices and charting. Finally, Novey says that *hiring an IM point person*, whose training enables him or her to speak the language of both biomedicine and CAM, increases the likelihood of successful institutional integration.

Vohra and colleagues (2005) conducted content analyses of notes from site visits to nine IM programs in North America. These programs, few of which were financially profitable, institutionalized two or more "pillars" of integration: clinical care, education, or research. Twelve key themes related to successful integration were identified: a small, flexible, low-cost start-up; hiring top clinicians; containing costs by hiring within; keeping the clinical component broad; keeping the research pillar focused; establishing and tracking evaluation benchmarks; documenting use; having the team in place before formally opening the clinic; keeping administration lean; making use of electronic record keeping; investing in high-end scalable information technology; and making sure that revenue-generating space takes priority.

In contrast to the focus on implementation factors for success, Barrett (2003) used a literature review to identify potential barriers and facilitators. He identified these facilitators of integration: belief in the effectiveness of CAM across the stakeholder groups (patients, providers, and health care decisionmakers); competition for patients; consumer demand; establishment of CAM's efficacy, cost-effectiveness, and lower risk; and, concomitantly, establishment of biomedicine's lack of efficacy and higher costs. In addition to the obverse of each of those factors, Barrett found that the following inhibit integration: fear of liability; reliance on habitual health-seeking behaviors; lack of availability of or insurance for CAM; and lack of standards, regulation, and credentialing for CAM providers.

In the United Kingdom, the Prince of Wales brought together a steering committee and working groups to examine the issue of integrative health care (Dalen, 1998). In this initiative, rigorous research into both CAM and conventional health care was seen as the basis for integration. In the UK, 22 integrative medical centers were surveyed and key components for success were identified (Dalen, 1998). The study concluded that CAM will thrive in mainstream health care where it satisfies an unmet need, but its successful integration will depend on the ability to address four key issues: attitudes of both CAM and conventional providers, evidence of effectiveness and safety, assurance of adequate training, and funding.

None of these recent studies, however, delineates what constitutes "successful" integration. So far, success is not the same as profitability. Whether these innovative centers and clinics are sustainable and develop long-standing referral pathways may hinge on their ability to identify, operationalize, and document not only evidence-based but economic, institutional, social, and individualized markers of success.

Consumer-Driven Integration

In one sense, patients were the first stakeholder group to achieve some form of integrative medicine. To a large extent, it is the patient who determines when to seek biomedical or CAM care and how this care is integrated into an overall health care plan. Few patients use CAM providers exclusively for their health care. Most CAM patients see a biomedical provider before or concurrent with seeking CAM care; only a small minority seek a CAM provider first (Paramore, 1997; Eisenberg et al., 1998, 2001; Ni, Simile, and Hardy, 2002; Barnes et al., 2004; Wolsko et al., 2004). For example, in the case of chiropractic care, over 80 percent of the patients retained the services of a biomedical physician (Kelner, Hall, and Coulter, 1980). However, it is significant that the majority of CAM patients do not disclose their use of CAM to biomedical providers (Eisenberg et al., 1993; Graham et al., 2005; Institute of Medicine, 2005), which increases health risks and potential iatrogenic effects.

Two national surveys of adults in the United States (Eisenberg, Kaptchuk, and Arcarese, 1993; Eisenberg et al., 1998) have shown that the use of CAM is extensive and increasing (from 33.8% of the population in 1990 to 42.1% in 1997). The 1998 study suggested that more patients visited CAM providers than primary care physicians and that the expenditures for these services (around $12 billion annually) were greater than for all hospitalizations in the United States during the same period (Eisenberg et al.). An increasing number of insurance companies cover CAM treatment (Pelletier, Astin, and Haskell, 1999; Pelletier and Astin, 2002). Patient use of CAM might suggest the emergence of an alternative paradigm of medicine, or it might be explained as a means of bridging the gap between the two worlds of medicine (Ullman, 1993; Jacobs, 1995).

Existing literature documents fairly consistent demographic patterns of CAM use, although the generalizability of these findings is problematic because of differences in how CAM has been operationalized. Women use both CAM and biomedicine with greater frequency than men. While it has been hypothesized that women's higher use of CAM reflects their social role as family caretakers, it is not known whether their own use of CAM results in overall higher CAM use in households. Caucasians report the highest frequency of CAM use excluding prayer, but recent studies suggest that lower CAM use among people of other ethnic/racial backgrounds may be the result of under-sampling (Graham et al., 2005). For example, Kim and Kwok (1998) documented that 62 percent of Native Americans saw indigenous healers as well as biomedical providers through the Indian Health Service. CAM use also appears to be greater in urban than rural areas (Barnes et al., 2004), while regional differences suggest higher CAM use in the Western United States, although this may reflect sampling biases (Wootton and Sparber, 2001). The most predictive demographic factors appear to be gender, age, and education level. The young and the old report lower frequencies of CAM use, with the highest usage across an inverse U from ages 18 to 65, and at higher levels of education (Eisenberg, Kaptchuk, and Arcarese, 1993; Eisenberg et al., 1998; Barnes, 2004). CAM users tend to be high-frequency users of health care in general, with two dominant pathways for CAM care-seeking: preventive health maintenance and treatment for chronic illness (Eisenberg, Kaptchuk, and Arcarese, 1993; Astin, 1998; Eisenberg et al., 1998). It has been hypothesized that once people use CAM, those who evaluate their outcomes positively may be more likely to increase their use of CAM for health maintenance purposes (Druss and Rosenheck, 1999; Sirois and Gick, 2002). However, as the Institute of Medicine report on CAM (2005) notes, the trajectory of how patients initiate and integrate biomedical and CAM modalities is not well understood.

Sociocultural Factors that Contribute to CAM and IM Use

The factors that have precipitated the rise in demand for CAM and IM are largely unknown and little researched. A speculative explanation (Coulter and Willis, 2004) for the phenomenon includes the aging population and the growing incidence of chronic illness and lifestyle-related morbidity rather than acute illness. In these areas, where biomedicine may be perceived to be less successful, CAM may appear to have much more to offer (e.g., the use of acupuncture for chronic pain). However, broad social shifts and significant personal life events appear to be most strongly associated with the increased CAM use, rather than patient dissatisfaction with biomedicine (Astin, 1998; Siahpush, 1998).

Siahpush (1998) demonstrates that values typically associated with postmodernism (e.g., challenges to the usefulness and meaning of globalizing bodies of scientific, medical, and technological knowledge and authority; a rise in consumerism; and a return to traditional and natural models of health) are most likely to predict favorable attitudes toward alternative therapies. These findings support sociological descriptions of how globalization affects individual values and is reshaping social norms and behaviors (Giddens, 2000). Similarly, Astin (1998) found that, in addition to the demographic factors associated with CAM use (e.g., female, higher education) and poorer health or chronic illness, personal factors also were predictors of CAM use. These factors might include a transformational experience that changed the person's worldview, a social commitment (e.g., to the environment, feminism), or an interest in spirituality or personal growth psychology. In addition, people report turning to CAM to avoid the adverse effects of pharmaceuticals and to learn more about nutritional, emotional, and lifestyle effects on health (Astin et al., 2000); because of a lack of confidence in biomedicine (McGregor and Peay, 1996); and from a desire for a holistic, nonreductionistic "ecology of health" (Micozzi, 2002).

These social shifts have significantly advanced the legitimacy of CAM. Traditionally, biomedicine could contain and restrict CAM by claiming to act in the public interest. As the consumer movement has gained strength and health care has become increasingly politicized, this approach has lost its legitimacy and legality. Consumers have demanded to act in their own interest, and legislation has made the restraint of trade illegal, even for medicine (Coulter and Willis, 2004).

Changing Medical Attitudes Toward CAM and IM

The significant number of hospitals that offer IM/CAM suggests that despite the long-term animosity in the United States of biomedicine toward CAM (Kaptchuk and Miller, 2005; Larson, 2005), over the past decade, biomedicine has moved from simply acknowledging the existence of CAM, to cooperating with it, to evaluating it, and finally to incorporating it. Whether this will effect a lasting change in bio-medical values and practice is yet to be determined (Ranjan, 1998), as is whether these changes will prove positive for CAM, biomedicine, or patients (Kaptchuk and Miller, 2005). And the changes are not limited to hospital-based IM/CAM. By 2000, 82 of 125 accredited U.S. medical schools included content related to CAM in their required curriculums (Wetzel et al., 2003). The number of medical schools that include CAM in their curriculums has been increasing annually since 1995, when CAM-related coursework was included at only 32 medical schools (Daly, 1995); the number increased to 42 in 1997 (Daly, 1997), 65 in 1998 (Bhattacharya, 1998), and 79 in 1999 (Bhattacharya, 2000). Most of these additions have occurred in schools of medicine, although some—like the one at Stony Brook (Blanchet, 1998)—brought together the schools of nursing, medicine, social welfare, dentistry, and health technology and management. However, acceptance of CAM courses in medical schools does not mean acceptance by all medical faculty. The faculty response to these courses has been mixed (Monson, 1995), and in many instances it is the medical students who have pushed for their inclusion (Wetzel, Eisenberg, and Kaptchuk, 1998). Practitioners who receive CAM training, especially those who are "dual-trained," are more likely to be open to and advocate for IM (Hsiao et al., 2006).

IM issues also can be found in medical practice. By 1998, it was reported that at least a dozen major medical schools had created treatment programs in integrative medicine. These efforts face unique problems (Coulter, 1999) but are probably facilitated where there is a commitment to include outcome assessments of CAM as an integral part of the program (Coates and Jobst, 1998).

Continuing education courses in CAM are being offered for medical physicians (Eisenberg, Kaptchuk, and Arcarese, 1993; White, Mitchell, and Ernst, 1996). With 40 percent of their patients having used CAM, medical physicians need to be conversant with the more common CAM practices, even more so if their patients are taking herbs, natural substances, and supplements that may interact with prescribed drugs. Astin and colleagues (2000) reviewed surveys of physician practice, referral, or interest in CAM and found wide variation in the attitudes of physicians. However, a meta-analysis of surveys on medical providers' attitudes showed that, overall, biomedical providers believed CAM to be moderately effective (Ernst, Resch, and White, 1995). Moreover, 50 percent of family physicians thought CAM represented legitimate medical practice (Berman et al., 1995); 60 percent reported making CAM referrals during a 12-month period (Borkan et al., 1994); and 68 percent of general practitioners reported some involvement with CAM during a previous seven-day period (White, Resch, and Ernst, 1997). As Barrett notes (2003), in addition to institutionalized integration, biomedical providers—like their patients—have been integrating medical paradigms, although much of this behavior remains undocumented or unpublished.

This shift toward CAM resulted in the 1998 establishment of the journal *Integrative Medicine: Integrating Conventional and Alternative Medicine*. In the first issue, the editor noted, "Paradigm shifts do not come easily in medicine" (Weil, 1998, p. 1). The journal has ceased to exist because, according to the editor, "[I]nterest in this area has become so keen that mainstream medical journals are not only accepting but actively encouraging submissions on CAM therapies and integrative strategies" (Weil, 2000, p. 1). A publication of the American Medical Association (AMA) (Fontanarosa and Lundberg, 1997) reported that *AMA Archives Journal* readers ranked alternative care among the top 3 of 86 subjects for AMA journals to address, and *Journal of the American Medical Association* (JAMA) readers ranked it 7th of 73 of the most important topics for publication in the journal.

Case Study of an Integrative Center

The literature establishes that a change has occurred in medical attitudes toward CAM, patient use of CAM, and the isolation of CAM from medical centers. The literature also documents the emergence of integrative medicine. What remains unclear, however, is what an IM center is, how and how much it is integrated within biomedicine, and the factors that facilitate or impede integration. Given our lack of understanding of IM, we need an in-depth exploration of the factors that inhibit or promote integration before vigorous quantitative research can be effectively conducted. Although reports exist on individual centers, no in-depth analysis of a center has been conducted.

This study addresses that gap in the literature. The study uses a mixed-methods approach to create an in-depth, systematic, qualitative, descriptive case study that delineates the key factors that inhibited and facilitated the establishment of an IM center in a nationally recognized hospital. In addition, the study is intended as an educational story that can guide those who seek to plan and create centers of integrative medicine.

Study Aims

A central aim of this five-year case study was to document the attitudes and behavior toward the center of selected groups (stakeholder groups), including hospital administrators and medical leadership; complementary and alternative medicine providers in the center; selected medical providers in the hospital; CAM providers in the adjacent area outside the hospital; and patients. The study also set out to document the extent to which CAM providers are integrated in the IM center, the hospital setting, and the larger community, and to establish the links among the stakeholder groups. We wished to identify the factors that contributed to and those that hindered integration of CAM in a hospital setting.

The study also compared the findings of this case study with those of other integrative medical units through a panel of experts drawn from such units.

The study was conducted over a five-year period beginning July 2001. Data were collected from February 2002 through December 2005. Data analysis and report writing were completed in December 2006.

Organization of the Report

The report is organized as follows. Chapter Two describes our analytic approach and the study design. Chapters Three through Five tell the story of the IM center's creation, operation, and ultimate demise. These chapters are organized chronologically. They draw on stakeholder interviews to provide essential material for understanding Chapter Six, which presents the evaluative findings from the stakeholder analysis. This analysis is organized around the themes that emerged from the interviews. Chapter Seven presents our conclusions: It identifies the principal facilitating factors and barriers to creating and sustaining a successful IM center and draws lessons for future efforts to integrate a CAM facility into a traditional hospital setting. In this report, we use the word "success" in two ways. The first is whether the center survived; in this sense, the center was not successful. But success can also refer to its achievements during its existence; in this sense, the center was successful.

CHAPTER TWO

The Study

Introduction

The emergence of centers of integrative medicine is well documented in the literature. Several points remain unclear, however. What is a center of integrative medicine? To what extent is it integrated with mainstream medicine? What factors are likely to facilitate or inhibit such integration? Although no in-depth independent analysis has been done of any single functioning center, we can study an integrated center by considering it a service delivery component embedded in a larger health system. Such systems can further be represented as a network of individuals (or stakeholders), and we can study how they interact with each other in different ways over time and space.

To analyze such a system, we draw on two research traditions: *stakeholder analysis* and *social network analysis*. Stakeholder analysis examines individuals' beliefs, behaviors, and vested interests (stakes) within and across groups. Social network analysis describes how the individuals interact with each other and with a larger system. Both analytic approaches recognize that people are members of groups with different objectives and interests, whose interactions are strongly influenced by group identity. Problems with integration can occur at both the individual and network levels.

Stakeholder Analysis

Stakeholders are presumed to have an agenda vis-à-vis the topic in question. Stakeholder analysis employs two basic approaches to determine the stakeholders' agendas (Weiss 1986; Hengstberger-Sims and McMillan, 1991). The first involves establishing conceptually the characteristics thought to constitute the agenda and then determining if the shareholders agree with those characteristics. This is normally done with structured questionnaires. The difficulty with this approach is establishing criteria that are general enough to cover the range of activities the stakeholder may wish to include but specific enough to distinguish one group from another. The researcher, in effect, creates an agenda by presenting characteristics the respondents might not have mentioned on their own. This approach generates objectively comparable data. It has been successfully used in the health system to understand emerging/evolving systems such as health maintenance organizations (HMOs) (Whitehead et al., 1989; Widra and Fottler, 1992) and urban-rural hospital alliances (Savage et al., 1992).

The second approach, called grounded theory research, sets aside the agenda and instead explores with the respondents, in their own words, what they perceive to be the important issues. By empirically documenting the opinions of the respondents, we can establish the agenda that is important to the stakeholders.

Qualitative researchers assume that the meaning of any observed behavior depends on the context in which it occurs, and they prefer "grounded" concepts and theories (Glaser and Strauss, 1967). In practical terms, this means approaching the field with a minimum of predetermined concepts and theories; those that are used must be amenable to constant revision as the research proceeds. The objective is to generate concepts that do not distort the phenomena under study (Van Maanen, 1979). When the focus is on operationalizing quantitative measures (particularly if this is done prematurely), it is possible to overlook relevant variables or oversimplify them (Mullen and Reynolds, 1978). Another advantage of grounded theory is that it is immediately available to the social participants—it is both comprehensible and self-obvious, because it is based on the participant's perspective.

In our case, the IM center brings together those who offer a service (CAM providers), those who are in a position to refer patients to a service (medical physicians), those who seek a service (CAM patients), and those who regulate integration (administrators). However each of these is locked into other systems with other stakeholders. For the CAM provider, it may be a particular profession, as in the case of chiropractors or acupuncturists, or it could be the community of CAM providers as a whole. If the CAM provider is a biomedical physician, the medical or hospital community could be part of his or her system. Each stakeholder will have a distinct stake in integrative medicine, and they may be in conflict.

Social Network Analysis

Individual stakeholders (both providers and patients) are linked together in complex webs of association. The analysis of such networks—social network analysis—provides a rich and systematic understanding of the relationships among people, teams, departments, or even entire organizations (Wasserman and Faust, 1994).

Integration can take various shapes and forms: (1) client-based links (client referrals and the sharing of client information); (2) program-based links, which can be formal (sharing staff, invited presentations, coordinating efforts) or informal (friendship networks, serving together on committees or boards, professional affiliations); and (3) indirect program links (funding sources, regulatory bodies, hospital hierarchies). The integration can be horizontal (among similar types of services) or vertical/functional (among varied but related services). Links can be analyzed in terms of organizational level (e.g., between agency heads, among frontline staff or intermediary program managers); scope of the linkage (i.e., the number of system members included in the relationship); how they are linked (informal versus formal relationships; written or binding agreements by authorized agents and informal network relations based on interpersonal familiarity and trust); degree of coupling; stability (as measured by length/duration of a relationship); and reliability.

A social network approach can be used to characterize systems of care and the extent and type of coordination and integration in these networks (Morrissey, Tausig, and Lindsey, 1985). Network analysis (Scott, 1991; Wasserman and Faust, 1994) allows various levels of analysis (Morrissey, Johnsen, and Calloway, 1997). It allows the researcher to determine the intensity and complexity of interdependencies among organizations, parts of organizations, or individuals (Van de Ven, 1976; Van de Ven and Ferry, 1980); and the degree of coordination among these organizations/parts. Network analysis has been used extensively to understand mental and physical health care systems from an organizational perspective (Morrissey, Tausig, and Lindsey, 1985; Wright and Shuff, 1995; Morrissey, Johnsen and Calloway, 1997).

An exploratory qualitative network analysis explores the multiple relationships among actors and groups. Like the "embedded" case study design described by Caronna, Pollack, and Scott (1997), the qualitative approach uses in-depth interviews to analyze links among social systems, individuals, organizations, and environments.

In our case, this approach helps us understand referral patterns, cooperation in planning, sharing of resources, coordination of services, and sharing of information (Eisenberg and Swanson, 1996; Jinnett, Coulter, and Koegel, 2002). In addition, the social network approach allows us to make sense of the structural (formal) organizational features as seen in a hospital organization chart as well as the informal relationships that people negotiate as they try to secure care for their clients. Once this range of relationships has been mapped, a more quantitative analysis can be applied.

Through the use of this dual framework, we can draw attention to the importance of stakeholder beliefs and attitudes as well as the network of relationships that are established in a social system. The approach allows us to delineate the important factors that facilitate or hinder integration.

[Note: Our research team collected the necessary data from the case study to conduct network analysis; however, the results of that analysis will be available in later publications.]

Study Design

Overview

We used a case study methodology to examine how a center for integrative medicine fits into a large hospital and community of stakeholders (Yin, 1984). Unlike large-scale survey methods, case studies are particularly effective for discovering the key factors that facilitate and inhibit desired outcomes, and understanding the process and mechanisms through which these factors interact (Patton, 1990). Case studies are one of the few techniques that provide in-depth information about how programs are working (or not working) in the larger social and organizational contexts in which they are embedded (Jinnett, Coulter, and Koegel, 2002).

As part of the case study approach, we drew on both qualitative and quantitative data collection and analysis techniques. Most of our data come from structured and semistructured interviews with six stakeholder groups: (1) key hospital administrators; (2) non-CAM clinicians in the hospital (attending physicians); (3) non-CAM clinicians in the community (private attendings); (4) CAM providers in the IM center; (5) CAM providers in the adjacent community; and (6) patients. In each interview, we asked people to report on their own experiences with CAM and the IM center, as well as their relationships with other persons and stakeholder groups associated with the center.

Qualitative data collection techniques have several key advantages over standard survey techniques: (a) respondents describe their experiences, beliefs, and choices in the way they think about them; (b) they are not limited to investigators' predetermined concepts and theories; and (c) they provide a more dynamic picture of processes and mechanisms that regulate social phenomena (Van Maanen, 1979; Patton, 1990; Miles and Huberman, 1994).

To complement our qualitative data, we also collected quantitative data from patient files and more structured patient questionnaires. By combining the many different stakeholder perspectives, we get a more nuanced and complete understanding of the evolution of the IM center and all the people who played roles in its growth and demise.

Finally, to place our case study in a larger framework, we held a one-day workshop with key personnel from other IM programs (successful and unsuccessful) throughout the country.[1]

In the following pages, we outline the research design and methods used in the project and briefly describe case study methodology, the study setting, and the stakeholder groups we included. We describe the organizational framework and its constituent parts: setup, research design, data collection techniques, data management, and selection of participants. Finally, we outline the analytic steps and discuss the generalizability of the results.

Study Setting

The hospital-based Integrative Medicine Medical Group (IMMG) is a multispecialty practice delivering primarily outpatient medical care in a collaborative fashion that coordinates complementary and alternative medicine with conventional western medicine. The IM center was established by the hospital in the summer of 1998 to coordinate integrative medicine activities throughout the hospital's health system. It was located in a community-based academic medical center with the full services of a teaching hospital. The IM center included two board-certified internists, an osteopath certified in family practice and geriatrics, two traditional Chinese medicine practitioners, a chiropractor, and a massage therapist. Services included western medical diagnosis and treatment, botanical medicine, nutritional counseling, mind-body interventions, acupuncture, Chinese herbal medicine, manual adjustments, craniosacral therapy, relaxation training, tai chi, limited homeopathy, and massage therapy.

Patients were seen initially by a biomedical physician, who coordinated their treatment plans. Close affiliations with other practitioners in the area extended the range of services to include chiropractic care,

---

[1]   The 12 panel members were chosen for their experience with or expertise in integrative medicine. Although their work does not form an integral part of the report, they provided a very powerful and efficient method of determining whether our case study shared elements found in other IM centers. The panel members and their affiliations are listed in Appendix A, along with a description of the panel's work. The workshop provided powerful confirmation that our results are valid for other institutions and not unique to the case we studied.

energetic healing techniques, classical homeopathy, Ayurvedic medicine, aromatherapy, and Rolfing. The IM center also assisted other academic departments that were interested in using CAM modalities or research in the application of these modalities to their patient populations. For example, a cardiothoracic surgery group investigated the use of acupuncture, massage, and guided imagery in the management of postoperative pain after coronary artery bypass grafting; and a multidisciplinary chronic fatigue study was planned with participation from the IM center and the departments of endocrinology, rheumatology, and psychiatry. The center also planned for regular participation in a diabetes outpatient program and the design of a coordinated research program. The center saw more than 1,000 patients from 1998 until 2001.

The IM center offered a unique opportunity to study the barriers and facilitating factors in the establishment of a center for integrative medicine in a mainstream medical facility. Because the experience was recent, the stakeholders had clear memories of the process that led to its establishment. For the most part, those who participated were still there at the time of the case study, so the issues and problems were still present or fresh in their minds. In addition, we were able to track the demise of the center, which ceased to exist as a formal entity in July 2001. The IM center provided an ideal site for an in-depth case study. Case study methodology produces information-rich descriptions of phenomena by bringing to bear multiple perspectives with multiple types of data from each perspective. Below we describe the stakeholders we interviewed and the types of data collected from each.

Sampling

Case study methodology relies on a two-step sampling procedure. Investigators first decide what case (or cases) they will examine (case-based sampling), and then decide what kinds of data they will collect from each case (within-case sampling). The power of case studies does not depend on the number of cases (in our case, n=1) but instead comes from the range and diversity of the within-case sample of people and data collection techniques. In this study, the case is represented by the integration of the IM center into its hospital setting and the within-case sampling is represented by multiple interviews collected from the various stakeholder groups.

Figure 2.1 shows the stakeholder groups and their relationship to the IM center.

The bulk of our data came from a stratified sample of stakeholder groups. The data from the stakeholders contributed to our analysis of their beliefs, attitudes, and behavior and to our network analysis of the relationships among the departments and other groups. In all the interviews, the ultimate focus was on the facilitators of and barriers to creating a center of integrative medicine. The following paragraphs describe the stakeholder groups; Table 2.1 gives the total participant count for each group.

Figure 2.1
Diagram of the Integrative Medicine Medical Group

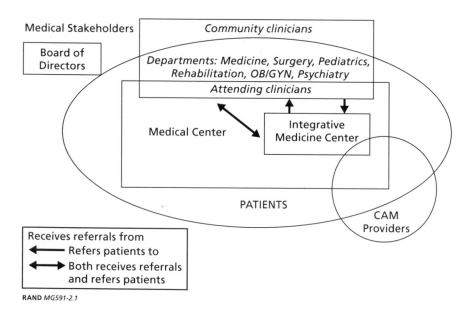

Table 2.1
Stakeholder Groups

Stakeholder	n
CAM community providers	41
IM Center patients	40
Attending clinicians	23
Community clinicians	21
IM center providers/staff	17
Administrators	16
CAM experts, donors, others	8
Board of directors	5
Total participants	171

a. Board members (n=5) included key members of the board, such as the chairperson and those who were identified as sponsors or supporters of the IM center.

b. Hospital administrators (n=16) included key personnel involved in establishing or setting administrative policies for the IM center. They came from throughout the medical setting and were key informants for the institutional history concerning the creation of the center, as well as current administrative goals and fiscal policies. The sampling of key informants was determined partly by their ability to inform (Johnson, 1990) and partly by the positions they held (Gilchrist, 1992).

c. IM center providers and staff (n=17) included all full- and part-time CAM providers who practiced in the center, as well as administrators and staff. We conducted individual face-to-face interviews with all members of the IM center. We used these interviews to explore their attitudes toward CAM and their beliefs about the center's mission, its place in the hospital, and its future. To increase our understanding of the network, we explored in detail the role each interviewee played in the center and the kinds and numbers of links that existed among center members.

d.   Attending clinicians (n=23) included those employed directly by the medical center. We obtained updated lists from the hospital personnel directory and broke them down by department and division. We selected mainstream providers who were most likely to be associated with CAM providers and the IM center because of the types of illness and disease they treated. We also interviewed providers in divisions that had referred patients to the IM center. For attending clinicians at the medical center, we first stratified by medical specialty. We selected providers with specialties in four areas in which the literature indicates strong patient use of CAM therapies: rheumatology, hematology/oncology, orthopedics, and obstetrics/gynecology (OB-GYN). For each of these specialties, we further stratified providers according to those who had referred patients to the IM center and those who had not. Referring clinicians were identified from abstracts of patient records and by providers in the IM center.

e.   Community clinicians (n=21) included private attending clinicians with hospital privileges at the medical center. These providers could act as a more removed source of referrals to the IM center; their role in the integration of the center into the community was unclear. As with attending clinicians, we used interviews to elicit data on community clinicians' attitudes, beliefs, and practices relative to CAM, and their links with the IM center.

f.   Community CAM providers (n=41) included CAM providers in the catchment area (the geographical area surrounding the hospital). The IM center had already identified a list of more than 700 providers who met this general criterion. CAM providers in the community can be an important base for referrals and an important source of legitimacy for an IM center—they have access to a patient population and a broad public whose attitudes they can influence. They also can function as providers in the medical center setting. On one level, they can be seen as competitors of the center; on another, they can function as a supportive community. We conducted individual interviews with these providers. We were particularly interested in interviewing providers who perform similar functions to those offered by the CAM providers at the IM center.

To select CAM providers in the community, we first stratified our sample into three specialty areas: chiropractic, acupuncture, and massage therapy/body sculpting. We interviewed providers identified by the IM center and asked these people to identify others they thought we should interview. This "snowball sampling" technique led us to add four more CAM modalities: naturopathy/herbalism, homeopathy, integrative medicine, and an "other" category that included a hypnotherapist, an art therapist, two yoga teachers, and a biofeedback specialist.

g.   Patients (n=40) included those who were seen at the IM center. Even when professional interaction on a personal level between medical and CAM providers is nonexistent, they are inextricably linked by their patients. We also used the center's patient files to identify referral patterns. We chose 40 patients to interview on the basis of four main presenting problems: pain, cancer, general health/checkups, and miscellaneous symptoms/conditions. The presenting problems and utilization data were abstracted from patient charts by center staff.

Although there are no strict rules for sample size for qualitative studies, they typically include 30 or fewer respondents (Patton, 1990). Some qualitative researchers recommend using at least 5 respondents to understand the essence of an experience and 30–50 respondents for interviews that cover numerous topics (Morse, 1994). In our case, we conducted 17 individual interviews with providers and staff of the IM center and 40 with patients. In addition, we interviewed 21 administrators, medical directors, and board members; 23 attending physicians; and 21 community physicians with admitting rights. For the provider stakeholder group outside the IM center, we interviewed 41 community CAM providers. We also interviewed eight respondents who were key CAM experts or donors. We tried to stratify informants across both mainstream medical and CAM specialties. We believe this sampling strategy was an excellent way to capture breadth of experience, and it increases our confidence in the generalizability of our results. The sample totals for all groups are shown in Table 2.1.

Data Collection Techniques

Data were collected using multiple methods (Miller and Crabtree, 1992), a strategy that yields higher quality case study results (Yin, Bateman, and Moore, 1983), then triangulated (Patton, 1990; Tashakkori and Teddlie, 1998) to increase the reliability and validity of the findings (Yin, 1984). Data were collected by multiple investigators (Lincoln and Guba, 1985; Patton, 1990) and were drawn from multiple points of view to reduce the influence of any single investigator (Edgerton and Langness, 1974). We used six interviewers, all trained in qualitative methods.

Although this was primarily a qualitative study, the combination of qualitative and quantitative techniques has long been recognized as a powerful research strategy (De Vries et al., 1992), especially for exploratory studies. We used quantitative data from patient records, patient intake surveys, and interviews of providers and patients.

These data from multiple sources allowed us to provide a descriptive account of the various stakeholders' attitudes, beliefs, and behaviors relative to CAM and the IM center.

    a.   Documents and archival research. We reviewed available documentary evidence relating to the center's policies and procedures: the business plan, organization charts, administrative documents (memorandums of agreement, statements of standard operating procedure, policy pronouncements), proposals, reports, minutes of meetings, letters, and other written reports pertaining to the creation of the center and its integration into the hospital and the adjacent community. These documents allowed us to begin piecing together a detailed portrait of the IM center.

b. Key informant interviews in the hospital. We used semistruc-
    tured interviews with key informants, including high-level
    administrators, IM center staff, and referring doctors. We
    covered the following topics: (1) historic factors surrounding
    the establishment of the IM center; (2) policies concerning
    the center and its integration in the hospital; (3) nature and
    determinants of structural relationships between mainstream
    providers and IM center providers; (4) procedures used to
    refer patients to IM center providers; (5) organizational and
    financial constraints that might contribute to the underuti-
    lization of IM center providers; and (6) characteristics of indi-
    vidual patients and providers that either facilitate or inhibit
    the use of IM center providers.
    All key informant interviews were conducted face-to-face by
    a team of two interviewers and were digitally recorded and
    archived. Recordings were transcribed verbatim.

c. Abstracting patient records. Hospital staff reviewed patient
    records in the IM center from its inception to identify (a) the
    referral source for the patient, (b) the primary diagnosis, (c)
    the providers seen, and (d) where (if anywhere) the patient
    was referred outside the IM center.

d. IM center patient surveys. To augment the patient data for
    sampling purposes, we mailed a survey to all IM center
    patients to gather the following data: demographic informa-
    tion; the reasons they sought treatment; how many times they
    visited; the types of providers they visited; and the treatments
    they received. From the responses, we chose 40 patients to
    interview.

e. IM center patient interviews and satisfaction scale. To col-
    lect more detailed information on people's experience with
    CAM in general and with the IM center in particular, we also
    interviewed a sample of patients by phone. Using informa-
    tion from the patient surveys, we selected persons who rep-
    resented the full range of presenting problems, such as pain,
    symptoms/conditions/syndromes, general health/checkup,
    and cancer patients seeking adjunctive treatment. To cap-

ture potential differences across illness types, we stratified this sample by high and low service utilization. We developed a semistructured interview protocol to determine how patients came to the IM center, what other options they had considered and tried, who influenced them in their decision-making, what apprehensions (if any) they had, and how they responded to and felt about the treatment they received. We conducted these interviews by phone to respect the patients' privacy and because some patients suffered from chronic illnesses and could not travel. As with the key informant interviews, all patient interviews were recorded and transcribed verbatim.

Patient interviews combined an open-ended set of questions and a closed-ended survey instrument—an ideal mix for situations in which there is only one chance to speak with a respondent (Bernard, 2006). In each topic area, open-ended questions were asked before closed-ended questions so as not to bias the respondent's answers (Becker, 1958; Spradley, 1979; Bernard, 2006). At the end of the interview, we asked patients to complete a satisfaction scale that was originally designed and tested for chiropractic patients (Coulter, Hays, and Danielson, 1994).

f. Community CAM provider interviews and "integratedness" (IM-32 scale). We used a similar semistructured interview protocol to interview outside CAM providers. During the first part of these interviews, we explored the providers' attitudes, knowledge, and experience related to complementary and alternative medicine in general. Whereas for patients we wanted to understand the salience of CAM in their lives, for CAM providers we were interested in the importance they placed on CAM as part of their patients' care.

In the second part of the interview, we explored the links (if any) between these outside CAM providers and the IM center. For providers, we wanted to understand what role (if any) CAM and the IM center played in the lives of their patients and in their medical practice. We were particularly interested in having mainstream providers identify the barriers they saw to CAM, and how CAM providers and clinics might make a difference, if they were not already doing so. Finally, we used the IM-32 scale, which captures the providers' attitudes and opinions about "integratedness" (Hsiao et al., 2005).

Multiple interviewers conducted face-to-face interviews to ensure that there was no single-interviewer bias. When possible, two interviewers were present for the interview. All interviews were recorded and transcribed. The interviewers also took field notes, which were typed and added to the transcriptions.

g.   Expert panel. Once our data analyses were near completion, we invited an expert panel of 12 members to review our preliminary results and give us feedback on these findings. The panel included a national representation of integrative medicine specialists and administrators, including several people who had set up similar centers in hospital environments. We treated the panel discussion like a large group interview; it was recorded and transcribed verbatim.

Data Management and Retrieval

To help synthesize the large amount of qualitative data this effort yielded, we used computer software designed specifically for narrative interviews and field notes (Pfaffenberger, 1988; Fielding and Lee, 1991). The software we used on this project was ATLAS.ti (Muhr, 1997–2004).

The data from the abstracting of patient records and all the survey data collected from patients and providers were entered into a relational database, which facilitated input into statistical packages as needed. We used SAS software to clean the data and produce results (SAS, 1999).

Analysis

We used multiple techniques to analyze our data. To analyze the key informant interviews (the bulk of our qualitative data) we used a multistep analysis. First, we coded the transcripts for specific time intervals to capture how the IM center evolved. We identified the following stages as the most important for understanding the rise and fall of the center: planning, setup, reorganization, and demise. For each stage, we decided when the period started and ended, and made these criteria explicit in our shared codebook. Next, coders read through the entire corpus of transcripts and marked text that corresponded to each period. To ensure that the coders were consistent, the project team addressed questions about particular quotes and reached consensus on them.

Second, we coded the transcripts for the kinds of stakeholders mentioned in the interviews. We knew we were interested in the role that different kinds of stakeholders played in the process, so we marked all texts where stakeholders such as the IM center director, the hospital CEO, the chief of the medical department, and others were mentioned. We followed marking and cross-checking procedures like those described above.

Third, we identified and coded 10 overarching themes we derived from the interviews. Each team member read through a sample of the interviews and identified various thematic categories that appeared. Themes are abstract (and often unclear) constructs that investigators identify before, during, and after data collection. They come from literature reviews, from the subjective experience of the investigators, and from the text itself. Each team member generated a thematic list, and then we met as a group and discussed our lists, arriving at a consensus about which 10 themes to follow. Our decisions were based on theme frequency and how important we felt the theme was in the development and demise of the center. Table 2.2 shows our list of overarching themes, with short descriptions. During the group meeting, we also started a thematic codebook. For each theme, we included a short description, inclusion and exclusion criteria, basic exemplars, and any exceptions to the rule.

Table 2.2
Themes

Overarching Themes	Short Descriptions
Academic Issues	Appointments, training, research
Administration	Business model, financial structure, legal issues, marketing/PR
Barriers	Issues that hurt the center
Competition/Referral Source	Internal and external competition and referral norms
Evidence Criteria	Evidence-based practice for CAM and biomedicine
Facilitators	Issues that helped the center
Leadership/Ownership	Staking ownership and champions of the center
Models	Types of IM models
Resistance to CAM	Types of resistance and unfounded expectation of resistance
Resources	Physical and staffing resources

Next, coders who were familiar with the interviews read all the transcripts and marked all examples they found of each theme. To ensure that we had as many instances of each theme as possible, coders were instructed to mark any instance that they felt was associated with a particular theme; when in doubt, they were to mark the segment. Marked segments ranged in size from a single sentence to several paragraphs.

We retrieved all marked segments for one theme and printed them out on separate pieces of paper. We randomly spread the printed segments out on a very large table and had team members read the segments and sort them into piles on the basis of similarities. The team members named each pile and described what each represented. After a lengthy group discussion, we identified the key sub-themes for each theme. Finally, we incorporated the sub-themes into our growing ATLAS.ti codebook, and two team members applied them to the marked text segments. This pile-sorting technique for identifying sub-themes is described by Lincoln and Guba (1985) and by Ryan and Bernard (2000).

Finally, we used the coded transcripts as the basis for our analysis and report writing. The first step in our writing strategy was to create a detailed description for each sub-theme—a kind of qualitative univariate analysis. To create the most comprehensive description possible, we retrieved all instances of each sub-theme, then used the text segments themselves to describe the range and central tendency of the abstract construct.

This was done by presenting both summary statements and exemplary verbatim quotes. These illustrative quotes served as prototypical examples of central tendency as well as exceptions to the norm.

The second step in our analysis was to examine how particular themes and sub-themes played out over time and across stakeholders—a kind of simple qualitative bivariate analysis. Here we used the search power of our text management software to identify text segments in which our sub-themes overlapped with different time segments and different stakeholders. For example, we pulled all text segments related to finance and then broke them down into each of the time periods. This helped us understand the role finance played as the IM center evolved.

We followed similar procedures for the more structured patient interviews. For each of the main questions in the interview protocol, we pulled all the unique responses and cut them out on separate slips of paper. We then used a similar pile-sorting technique to classify responses into fundamental categories.

For the structured section of the patient interviews, patient satisfaction, and provider integrated scale information, we entered the quantitative data in a spreadsheet and used standard univariate and bivariate analysis techniques to examine the range, central tendency, and distribution of responses within and across types of respondents.

Although our analysis is primarily exploratory and descriptive, and is not designed to formally test hypotheses, its scientific merit comes from our examination of the variation within and across informants, stakeholders, time, and place. By collecting information from such a diverse range of sources and using multiple analytic techniques to identify patterns, we have been able to systematically describe the empirical and theoretical factors that may contribute to the success and failure of IM centers.

CHAPTER THREE

Creation and Development

We tell our story chronologically in three phases: first the creation, then the operation, and finally the demise of the center. Like any complex story, this one has twists and turns, and resists reduction to a simple plot. This is not a story of either success or failure but one of successes and failures. It is a story from many perspectives—people who have quite different interpretations of events. It is a personal story, one that could be told as a story of individuals. It is also a partial story: No research methodology can hope to capture the whole story in complex social systems.

Because of the significance of the first phase—planning the IM center—we describe it in detail.[1] We have divided the center's creation into three phases: the initial impetus, the task force, and the business model.

Initial Impetus

The IM center's beginning had two major actors: the hospital's board of directors and the Department of Medicine. By 1996, members of the Department of Medicine were well aware of the results of studies by David Eisenberg that identified three major issues with regard to CAM in the United States. First, a lot of people were using it; second,

---

[1] See time line in Appendix B.

they were spending a lot of money on it; and third, many of them were not telling their medical physicians about their CAM use.

The landmark study by Eisenberg, Kaptchuk, and Arcarese (1993) documented high rates of out-of-pocket CAM use by a significant proportion of the U.S. population. This study laid the foundation for attempts to incorporate CAM into a hospital environment. Part of the motivation was economic: The report made the business case for integrating CAM and triggered a vision of patients with cash in hand flocking to a medical center for CAM treatments. The economic incentives were augmented by the medical culture's core value of "doing no harm" to patients, and physicians' basic responsibility to do all they can to protect the health of their patients. If patients were "voting with their feet" by using CAM but not revealing that use to their biomedical providers, the potential was perceived as high for an iatrogenic impact as a result of herb-pharmaceutical interactions of CAM and medical procedures. Moreover, CAM represented an opaque knowledge base (e.g., a "black box") for these professionals, who pride themselves on their medical knowledge and training. Their patients were seeking treatments they knew little about, with illness models that did not fit their traditional pathogenic or physiological medical models.

Personal contact with patients and colleagues who sought and championed CAM care became another incentive to learn more about it.

> I think members of our board, maybe members of our medical staff, have had personal experiences around this and wanted to know where [the hospital]—which is effectively a full-service organization—would want to go with that. [Administrator P12][2]

---

[2]   Throughout the report, quotes are referenced by the type of respondent and a unique identifier that begins with the letter P. Respondents are grouped into the following general categories for the sake of anonymity: board of directors, administrators (some of whom are medical doctors), hospital providers, IM center providers, IM patients, community CAM providers, and experts in the CAM and IM fields.

It was assumed that many of the hospital's patients, and possibly staff members, were using CAM, but that the former were not telling their hospital-based providers. For the patients, this raised the issue of the interactive effects that might occur between CAM treatments and hospital-provided care. It also suggested a potential source of revenue that the hospital was not tapping and an opportunity for the hospital to provide a highly desired service for its patients. Some board members were already enthusiastic supporters of CAM, with spouses who were using it as well.

These shifts in the kind of care patients and colleagues were seeking presented moral and economic dilemmas for the hospital's executives, who saw an economic opportunity but may not have wanted the hospital to be associated with CAM. However, given the reported high rates of CAM use, exploring CAM was scientifically and economically attractive to these executives.

Exploration would enable biomedical professionals to test the validity of some CAM approaches. In addition, CAM held the promise of being an effective means of health promotion and source of low-cost, noninvasive modalities to contain escalating health care costs, which are a key concern of the dominant health services model of managed care. Moreover, providing CAM would enable the hospital to draw from this apparently vast yet institutionally untapped revenue stream.

Many of the hospital staff believed that the institution would be an appropriate test site for CAM and that they could apply scientific methods to this field. In doing this research, they would be in a position to support or refute the claims made for CAM.

Managed care also figured prominently. People were aware of health economics and knew how much money they were paying out of pocket for alternative medicine. There was an interest in understanding whether providing access to alternative medicine might be a strategy that would allow health care costs to be maintained within a capitated model. To the extent that alternative treatment could be less expensive, it could be a strategy to manage costs.

The Board of Directors' Role

Some members of the board supported the initiative, but the important fact was that it was perceived among the medical staff of the hospital as a "board initiative."

While the board is mandated to set policy and raise money, a board member may advocate for a program and foster a positive outcome during the approval process. A positive climate for a new program is enhanced if the program is positioned as serving the hospital's broad mandate of being at the forefront of innovation (leader of the pack).

> I think it's fair to say that it would be very unusual for the board to mandate the establishment of a program. We're trying to be responsive to the community's needs, and we should have systems in place to measure the community's needs, but not say, "How about this or that?" We might say, "Take a look at this, see what you think." We wouldn't say to them, "Put this program into effect on January first." . . . We're really a policy and fundraising board. So we try and keep out of it, not pushing too hard, but being helpful. [Board P22]

> Full board support for a program is not necessary.

> It depends upon their ability to sell the rest of the membership. If they have some good strong points that they can bring up and discuss with management, administration, and the other board members, they could perhaps bring it back for discussion and open it up and see where it goes again. [Board P26]

Board Approval Process for New Programs

The IM center plan was shepherded through the approval process by two of the hospital's vice presidents and a board advocate. The process included reviews by an initial planning committee, the Medical Executive Committee (MEC), and, finally, the board of directors.

> The Medical Executive Committee comprises the department heads, senior management, and physicians. They made a presen-

tation to the Medical Executive Committee, which is the end-all with boards that present this. When they give their blessing, it means the highest level of the hospital and the highest level of the medical group are in agreement about the direction they want this to proceed, or at least what they've been instructed. [Administrator P34]

Any new program has to have a business plan and financial analysis to get board approval. If it is a totally new program, it has to go through the board of directors.

So this program was taken through all of the steps of the normal routine for starting a program. It was approved by the board of directors to be developed. And there was actually a great deal of support for the medical center to get involved in providing these alternative methodologies. Because, let's face it, in California, I would say that a majority of the people here use some type of alternative medicine. [Administrator P71]

In the context of the hospital's faltering profits, the assumption that the center would be a moneymaking venture, drawing from a new revenue stream, bolstered its chances for approval. Profitability, however, is not the sole determinant in the approval process or in the sustainability of a program over time. In fact, most of this hospital's programs are not profitable. If a program is in the red but can be positioned as serving community needs, it may be retained. In the case of the IM center, the board was influenced by the fact that so many people, including the hospital's own patients and members of the community, were taking advantage of various forms of CAM. So the hospital was being responsive to community needs. The board also saw a big financial opportunity in this endeavor.

Board Climate

Although the board members claim it was not their mission to establish a program, at least one member was a strong and effective advocate for the program. The MEC's approval of the CAM program's business plan further influenced the board's review process.

They probably were seeing practitioners, having a little acupuncture themselves, so they were quite familiar with what was happening. We were trying to figure out, was it something that we should be getting involved with at the time. . . . And then the big thing was [the approval by the MEC], which is made up of the heads of the departments and all the senior people and the physicians; when they examined and approved it, that certainly gave us the confidence that we could try it. We weren't going to do it without their approval, and that was the big step—getting that group of regular, scientifically based physicians to approve this try. [Board P22]

Influence of Hospital Culture on the Board

The board was influenced in part by one of the hospital's core mandates, formally codified through branding with a motto that captured the idea of "leading the pack." This ethos indicates a proactive stance toward exploring, developing, and promoting novel medical programs, such as integrating an IM center into a hospital setting.

We always like to think we're on the leading edge of medicine. We're very proud of [this hospital]. We felt if we could make it work here and do it in a way that was scientifically based, that would be a breakthrough. We could kind of lead the way, because we liked the idea. Maybe being from [this hospital] we think that way—showing other people how to do it. We thought we had the ingredients to do it. [Board P22]

Along with innovation, the hospital's organizational culture values its roots in the community, responsiveness to community needs, intellectual openness, and entrepreneurship. The idea of a CAM program touched on each of these values. It required the hospital staff to be intellectually adventurous by being open to different medical models. It fostered attentiveness to the perceived community needs of patients who were using CAM. The idea of integrating biomedicine with CAM and potentially tapping into a lucrative revenue source was well suited to the institution's entrepreneurial focus.

This is an academic medical center with community hospital roots, as opposed to our friends at [X or Y universities]. And that creates a very different dynamic, and a very different culture, in terms of openness and in terms of entrepreneurship. There's a sense of entrepreneurship within this institution. The realistic side of it as well, I think, [is] that the medical staff didn't feel that this was going to be economically threatening to them. Being very candid, if they felt this was going to be economically threatening, they may not have been as open-minded. [Administrator P27]

The Task Force

The outcome of this initial phase was the establishment of a task force, which undertook two assignments: It sent a small group to observe and learn from existing centers of integrative medicine or CAM in hospitals, and it developed a business plan.

And so, the first thing I did is I went to our CEO and I said to him, "I'm interested in looking into this and possibly developing a program. What do you think?" And he said, "Great. Why don't you go develop a task force and see what you can do?" And he said to speak to the chairman of the board just to make sure, because this is a fairly controversial topic for a conservative medical center. So I spoke to the chairman of the board. And the first thing he said to me was, "What took you so long?" So I had buy-in at the top of the institution for the program. [Administrator P6]

The task force was multidisciplinary. It included key players but also persons perceived as potential threats or necessary allies. Two of the key players were physician administrators, one was a successful IM practitioner, one represented the CEO's office, and at least one was a board member. Over time, the task force also included a pharmacist, a pathologist, surgeons, and an OB/GYN provider.

There were two schools of thought among the hospital staff about the impetus for the task force. One was that it came from the board.

I believe the real impetus for the program started at the board level. I think there was an interest by our board of directors, which led to its own internal procedures, to the creation of a task force to examine the implications of the study and the feasibility of developing such a capability here at [the hospital]. [Administrator P12]

Another view is that the impetus came from the medical director. At the same time, the hospital began to hold educational sessions and meetings about CAM in the hospital.

We started having meetings and we had lectures, and had to have the Chiropractic College come in. We had a variety of presentations to bring us up to speed . . . so there's a lot of background work and maybe presentations every week to different members of the [hospital] staff. So I made a bunch of presentations to the board of directors, I made presentations to the MEC, to the Medical Advisory Committee, to different departmental advisory committees, to nurses . . . and kept everybody abreast of this and had a lot of discussions with the MEC. And then we met a lot with pharmacy about the herbs. [Administrator P6]

The buy-in was so successful that the task force had to turn away colleagues who wanted to serve on it. Task force members discovered that many physicians were already either using or practicing CAM.

One physician phoned up and said, "You know, I've been doing this quietly for years and I haven't told my colleagues because they'd have shunned me." [Administrator P6]

The strong interest in a CAM program among hospital physicians suggested that the assumption of large-scale resistance was misguided. With the exception of some older staff and specialists, the proposal for an IM center encountered little explicit in-house resistance.

As you might imagine, there was a lot of resistance to this from some of the specialists in the older medical staff, and there were younger members of the medical staff who were very much interested in this. But, by and large, what happened is the medical staff said, "Look, we've known you for a long time, you're a traditionally trained physician, we know with your research background and everything else that you aren't going to lead us too far astray. And if you say you're going to watch over this, then we'll trust you and let you go ahead and do this." And one of the advantages we had is that this was a top-down program rather than a bottom-up program, so it had a lot of support. [Administrator P6]

The task force also reviewed internal staff utilization of the key CAM service covered by Blue Cross at that time—chiropractic—to determine how hospital employee use of CAM compared with the national data cited in the 1993 Eisenberg, Kaptchuk, and Arcarese publication. The task force followed the traditional academic process by reviewing the literature first. It also looked at hospital employee population utilization data from Blue Cross, the hospital's insurance carrier. They discovered that the percentage of their own employees who were seeing CAM providers as part of their benefit package mirrored the use in the general population (25–35%). However, these figures were the only local data they had about the need for CAM services.

Following this cursory review of the use by health care workers of services covered by their insurance policies, the task force members contacted other medical clinics and academic medical centers with CAM/IM components and arranged site visits. The information they gathered from these visits allowed them to compare different models, revenue structures, liability concerns, and clinical interfaces. Through this process, they identified a potential niche market and developed a plan for an integrative medicine outpatient clinic.

We went around the country talking to people; gathering information about their experience, their structure, pitfalls, and whatnot; and assembled those data, and came back to the committee with our experience and proposals for different kinds of models and approaches. . . . We came up with an integrative model. [Administrator P8]

The task force came to the conclusion that it would not support a model of CAM alone, because the members did not think the hospital could compete with the numerous and varied CAM practitioners in nearby communities. The task force wrote a report about the site visits.

> We did a business plan that we presented to the board in June 1997 . . . the task force took some time coming to that model. We wanted to understand what happened to other institutions, where they were going with [CAM] and so on. . . . We found out how they were constructed and what their issues were. At that time, too, there was a question as to how much of this would be payable by insurance versus how much would be cash-and-carry business. So there was a liability question attached to that. We presented different models to the committee, and the committee supported the model we were proposing, which was an integrative model that would be primarily outpatient. It's generally an outpatient practice, but with an acknowledgment that there might be need for consultation and treatment on the inpatient side. [Administrator P8]

It was hoped that identifying a niche market with a "sweet spot" (a model that integrated CAM and biomedicine) would help the center avoid the pitfalls the task force had learned about during site visits. Some programs were housed in substandard environments and treated like biomedicine's unwanted stepchildren. For the task force, the "going-in premise or belief" was that alternative medicine had its place; traditional medicine had its place; and they should be bought together in a way that enabled movement of the patient from one modality to the other as seamlessly as possible.

Developing the Model[3]

The proposed model sought to integrate the best of both medical paradigms while ensuring that patients would receive this benefit within the safety net of a prestigious, traditional medical center. It had a tripartite clinical, research, and education design, with a research component that would test and advance CAM through an evidence-based approach. This would allow the hospital to patent and profit from some of its findings, while the teaching component would disseminate the research and clinical findings, and train future CAM/IM practitioners. This model would ensure that the center would meet the institutional mandate of leading the pack.

> We wanted to put together a model that would have patients be evaluated by a process that would blend eastern and western medicine together and come up with the best combined program for the patient. . . . We wanted somebody who could understand the clinical issues and wouldn't be treating prostate cancer with acupuncture, and would know to make a correct referral, make the appropriate triage decisions, and know what kind of referral to make for either western medicine or alternative medicine. That was the model . . . . Also, we didn't think that from the point of view of benefiting the literature, which was part of the other criteria that we were looking to do, that simply replicating what other people could do . . . would be helpful. We thought from the point of view of who we were as an institution, simply having alternative medicine out there alone wouldn't mesh well with the rest of what we did. [Administrator P12]

From the beginning, the administration recognized problems with this proposed model. Territorial issues are not unique to this center; they can be found whenever an innovative program threatens specialty

---

3   Eventually, three models were developed for the center. The first, developed by the task force, we call the *proposed model*. It was approved by the board and the Medical Executive Committee. The second model was developed by a member of the task force and the first director of the center, and was rejected by the senior administrators. We call it the *revised model*. We call the third model the *implemented model*.

barriers. The problem the administration saw with integrative medicine was that it is very hard in the politics of the hierarchy of medical institutions to integrate one program into the numerous units in the hospital. For an integrative approach, administrators had to overcome the hurdles of territorial jurisdictional issues. Those involved in the center thought the integration could be achieved through patenting remedies, doing clinical work, publishing, and eventually serving an educational role in the institution. The latter would involve bringing change agents together to educate them.

A niche market or "blended model" approach was thought to be potentially most effective. It would foment cultural exchange and change among both biomedical and CAM/IM practitioners. However, to increase the appeal to hospital physicians, the exchange process would be one-way. The proposed model defined its staff as "consultants" to whom hospital staff could refer a patient, knowing that the patient would be "returned" to the referring physician.

> We knew that up front there might be a concern about referrals. So we had designed the practice, and we had communicated the practice as not being one that was interested in long-term primary care medicine. Referrals that might be made by physicians would be returned back to that physician. The specific issue would have been addressed on a consultative basis and sent back, or treated on an agreed-upon plan between the primary care physician and [the IM] group. That was the plan. [Administrator P13]

The task force considered three possible models for the center, which at this point was called the Complementary Medicine Program[4]: (1) the university model, which combines research, teaching, and service; (2) a partnership with an existing CAM clinic; and (3) a for-profit clinic within the hospital. Initially, the task force pursued the second option by attempting to recruit a CAM provider with a highly success-

---

[4] In the initial discussion it was conceived as a center of alternative medicine. It later became a center of complementary medicine and ultimately a center of integrative medicine, or IM center.

ful clinic and bring it into the hospital, or form some sort of relationship with it. This attempt was unsuccessful.

Among the various stakeholders, the following key assumptions underlay the initial venture:

- Patient demand existed for these services.
- The rate of referral to such a clinic would be high.
- The venture would be profitable.
- Because of the reputation of the institution, the center would be successful.
- "If we build it they will come"—that is, the center would generate its own demand for services.
- Considerable opposition would come from some of the medical staff.

The task force developed a business plan, the board reviewed it, and the IM center was launched. The model that was implemented was a for-profit clinic, but it was set up as a separate entity from the hospital as a professional corporation. (As we explain in Chapter Six, this legal decision had major ramifications for the center.)

Along with these assumptions went a corresponding belief about the need to provide patients with greater choice in health services. The hospital, like any institution, does not exist in a social vacuum. Hospitals are sensitive to pressure from patients as consumers who expect to be able to choose from an array of medical options to meet their needs.

> The initial drive was, this is something we believe that the public wants. In this consumer-driven health care system, the public wants to have more access to these types of modalities and began to demand more access to those modalities. So, if you're a large institution like us, you would say, let's make sure we have a lot of things for them to pick from. But on a cost-per-unit-of-service basis, it was extremely high. [Administrator P66]

In the past, a hospital's losses could be made up through cost-shifting. In the current medical and insurance climate, this is accomplished by diversifying payer types; maximizing high-profit spin-offs, such as surgeries and outpatient tests; and marketing to ensure a flow of new patients and high patient volume.

> [You] really intensely focus your payer mix on areas where you can actually start to pay for some of this . . . [because] every patient doesn't pay for themselves. It's not like the old days where all the Medicare costs got shifted onto insured patients, but we know that some services in this hospital lose money. Pediatric makes no money. Endocrinology loses money. They don't do any procedures. Surgery makes money for the hospital. So you've got to realize, okay, what can we do, what's a reasonable amount of cash flow to make this thing work, and what's our net loss accept-ability within the system? And then, all the ways we can make up for it with outpatient [services]. Can we bring new business to the hospital? New business is huge. They love new business, because that's where they can measure the benefit of a program easier than anything else . . . if you can show that you brought in 100 new patients a month through the hospital . . . then the hospital starts saying, "Hey, this is a pretty good deal. We like that." [Hospital Provider P16]

Changing the Model

After the task force presented the model for a research-driven IM center to the Medical Executive Committee, an important shift in empha-sis occurred. Senior administrators focused on the clinical component rather than the research component, believing that the former would serve as a financial "engine," generating funds to support the research and education programs.

> The model for this wasn't driven by the profit motive, or even to make it solvent . . . . We had a general understanding that . . . it is research, and that it was up to the doctors to generate more research and once they got the research going, they would look at the clinical practice and they would be able to share time doing research and then have their clinical practices on the side. That

was the primary basis for it . . . . There was miscommunication on a lot of people's part . . . they thought that they would get enough either NIH grants or industry support to be able to fund some of the clinical activities and explore those on a case-by-case basis . . . somebody who could bring in drug trials [or the equivalent for] herbs and concoctions . . . . That was the presentation to the MEC, which is the end-all with boards that present this. So when they give their blessing that means the highest level of the hospital, the highest level of the medical group, are in agreement that that's the direction they want this to be proceeding. [Administrator P34]

A major change in the model soon followed. Given the board's mission to protect the hospital's limited seed funds, the administration (in contrast to the MEC) made it clear that the clinical component should generate profits.

We try to follow a pretty rigorous business planning process here. We don't have a lot of money, institutionally, to throw around. In an area like this, we have a relatively insignificant amount of seed capital that I felt we were really able to put into it. When I say relatively, I think probably a couple hundred thousand dollars. We're a billion-dollar organization. In the course of the development of that budget, one of the things that from a business-planning standpoint was then and remains key to the success of this, at least in this geographic area, was a successful clinical patient treatment enterprise. [Administrator P27]

The story of the morphing of the business plan follows a circuitous path; one that had major ramifications on the form the center finally took as a significantly revised and modified business model was enacted. Three models were created. The first, the *proposed model*, was submitted for approval to the board and the MEC. When they were unable to implement this model, the first director of the center developed a second model, the *revised model*. The senior administrators rejected this model and created the *implemented model*.

Initially, the task force hoped that an established CAM provider with a highly successful clinic could be persuaded to bring the clinic into the institution, along with the patient base. When that person declined the offer, a task force member was identified as the top candidate to direct this enterprise because of his medical, CAM, and business expertise. This person was hired as a consultant, although, functionally, he was head of the Complementary Medicine Program. His first responsibility was to set up the internal and external administrative processes for credentialing CAM providers. He was also charged with setting a research agenda and developing ties with other departments for joint projects.

After the credentialing process was successfully completed, a disagreement about the second model began to emerge. This fissure was between the head of the medical department, who favored a university model that would follow the hospital's normal mode of staffing new programs with world-renowned experts, and the more practical vision that the institution had to grow the program as quickly as possible.

It became clear that the business objectives of the task force plan were not achievable, and some administrators realized that it was going to take a long time to establish the IM center. They recognized that IM providers could not treat as many patients as the task force had projected; for example, an acupuncture treatment takes 40 minutes, far longer than the traditional physician encounter.

> How many patients get a 40-minute visit in an outpatient facility? Doesn't happen. On the other hand, you can't bill [it] out as a surgical procedure. With even a minor surgery, you can get a big reimbursement. So you're kind of stuck in a lot of different ways. [Administrator P36]

Concerned about the increasingly limited funds available to the clinic, the head of the program, proactive board members, and the IM physician the task force hoped would head the fledgling IM center came up with an alternative business plan. The clinic would be located outside the hospital and would be part of a consortium with local hospitals. This would enable the clinic to draw on a broader patient base and diversify payer types. Once it was set up, the hospital would contract with it. The clinic also would act as a consultant for other hospitals and groups that were interested in setting up IM clinics.

Unfortunately, the senior administrators and medical personnel at the hospital interpreted this new business plan as usurping the program to shop it around to other hospitals and medical centers. This led to a parting of the ways between the head of the medical department and the first director who had proposed the model. The latter left the hospital. It is unclear whether the implosion of the first unworkable business model and the failure of the second model led to the creation of the model that was implemented; that is, whether the final plan was partially a result of being "burned" by the earlier attempts.

Summary

Several factors provided the main impetus for the creation of the IM center. There was evidence of substantial consumer demand for complementary and alternative medicine. The hospital's chief of medicine was a strong advocate for the center, and there was a perception of strong support from the board of directors.

A respected task force compiled a report based on the literature and on site visits to other IM centers, and proposed a model for the center. The board and the Medical Executive Committee approved the initial plan. Under the consultative model, the center would be able to work in harmony with preexisting hospital programs, providing specialty services and not primary care. Such a program was congruent with the hospital's missions of initiating innovative programs and meeting community needs. An organizational home in the hospital foundation was proposed to house the new IM center.

CHAPTER FOUR

Implementation and Operation

In this chapter, we describe the implementation of the chosen model and present a profile of the center at the peak of its operations, between 1998 and 2001.

Introduction

Running the Center: Administrative Structure

The center's administrative structure is shown in Figure 4.1. The center was located in a foundation that existed in the hospital. The foundation (originally modeled after the Howard Hughes Medical Research Foundation and the Gladstone Foundation) was instituted by the board to give programs more flexibility. It provides an umbrella for two local but geographically noncontiguous medical groups and offers shelter from the Stark regulations[1] by housing hospital-affiliated programs as physician-owned professional corporations (PCs).

---

[1] The 1989 federal mandate (Omnibus Budget Reconciliation Act of 1989, Section 1877)—originally drafted by Representative Pete Stark (D-CA) and commonly referred to as the "Stark regulations"—was intended to ensure that physicians do not have a direct or indirect means to benefit financially from referring patients for services, procedures, prescriptions, supplies, or equipment. In essence, it is an anti-kickback rule. Amended in 2001 to prohibit unnecessary referrals of Medicare patients, the current statute has broad exemptions, including all academic medical centers. This "final rule" "generally permits physicians to refer to entities that they have a compensation relationship to, as long as the compensation paid to the physician is no more than would be paid to someone who provided the same services but was not in a position to generate business for the entity." (U.S. Department of Health and Human Services, 2001)

Figure 4.1
Administrative Structure

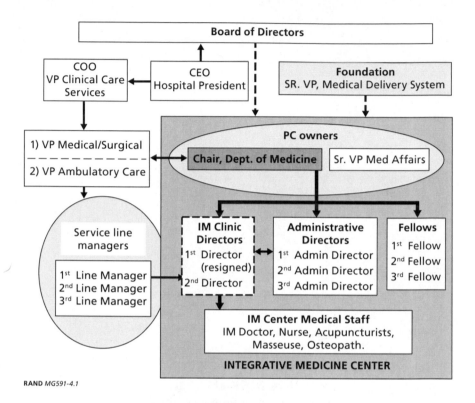

RAND *MG591-4.1*

They have some tax benefits and there are certain freedoms in operation as long as you follow the directions of the IRS. It's a very good format. [Board P14]

Initially, a CAM program was proposed that would be housed in the hospital's ambulatory care clinical programs. Ultimately, however, the center was not established in the medical center of the hospital's broader "health system." Instead, it was made part of the "physician delivery network" (versus the medical center or education and research), with four other groups also housed under the foundation. There was no direct link between the foundation and the IM center; that is, the foundation did not initiate the creation of the center. The link was that a hospital executive who was trying to assist in the development of a Department for Alternative Medicine was knowledgeable about how the foundation worked as an administrative and legal structure.

As a consequence of the center being housed in the foundation, the center director was technically not part of the hospital.

> The director of the center was, in fact, not employed by the hospital but employed by the PC, which was owned by two individuals. The reason was that laws state that a hospital cannot employ a physician in the practice of medicine. [IM Provider P11]

Incorporating the Center

The original plan was to establish the IM center as a cash-only business that provided services for the outpatient program in the Department of Medicine. Subsequent decisions regarding the administrative structure of the center were driven by a combination of regulatory constraints and potential incentives. Of the multilevel legal constraints, federal regulations regarding the corporate practice of medicine were the key factors in determining the center's initial administrative structure.

A professional corporation (i.e., Physician X Medical Group d/b/a Integrative Medicine Medical Group, Inc.) was established to deal with these restrictions, as it put the center legally at arm's length from the hospital. Other incentives to incorporate were to create a protective environment for innovation and for the anticipated financial remuneration for the corporation and the providers, such as above-scale salaries and bonuses tied to patient volume. Additional legal constraints were associated with the decision to incorporate, including regulations regarding the sale of pharmaceuticals, state-level billing codes, and hospital-level regulations mandating the acceptance of Medi-Cal and Medicare.

The hospital, which does not have tax-exempt status, comprises three business units: the hospital, teaching and research, and medical delivery. The impact of legal constraints on the IM center's administrative structure was most central to the last. The hospital's medical delivery network includes the medical group and an association of independent physicians. This association includes 750 nonhospital physicians. Because hospitals cannot own physician practices, approximately 80 physicians belong to the medical group. This entity, which buys and runs medical practices, is exclusively contracted to the hospital foundation.

> This is how the Hospital can buy practices. That's why this whole Foundation is here, because hospitals can't be in the corporate practice of medicine. There are very stringent laws against this. In the 90s, a lot of hospitals, in an effort to make sure that physician and patient practice bases were attached to them without violating the Stark regulations, they did something that created a Foundation, which bought doctors practices, and then took those same doctors, or hired new doctors, and or both, which created a Medical Group, so that those doctors then provided medical services to those patients. Then those practices got rolled up into a larger group with alleged savings in management and overhead. And this group pretty much admits only to [the hospital]. [IM Provider P5]

So the foundation provided the IM center with a shelter from regulatory oversight in general and the Stark regulations in particular. The rationale for incorporating was that the center would have a protective environment so the hospital did not have the burden of full regulatory oversight. It meant that the center would not be burdened excessively by bureaucratic rules, by what could and could not be done in the hospital; for example, by the rules of the Joint Commission on Accreditation of Healthcare Organizations (JCAHO).

It is noteworthy that this particular hospital is the only hospital of its *kind* in the state of California that falls under the rule preventing ownership of medical clinics.

> The rule exempts state-owned institutions, county-owned institutions, other government institutions, and, I think, university hospitals. So we're the only hospital of our stature in the state that falls under a rule that no one else of equivalent stature goes by. That has far-ranging political and economic implications for us,

our physicians, our relationship with others. Unlike other hospitals in medical school settings, where they can just hire physicians to provide that service, we couldn't do that. [Administrator P12]

While this private hospital is less politically entrenched than a university-based medical school and, therefore, able to encourage and support innovation, its lack of formal university or government affiliations makes it vulnerable to the most stringent interpretations of the Stark regulations.[2]

The normal process would be to develop a program and bring in full-time staff who are hired by the medical center. The programs include the teaching, research, and clinical arms; patients, seen on medical center property, are covered by medical center insurance. Such a program would potentially fall under the Medical Executive Committee rules and regulations and oversight. However, the model chosen in this case was to create a physician-friendly professional corporation, a special corporation of which the chief medical officer (CMO) and the chief financial officer (CFO) of the hospital would be the owners.

Financial Incentives for Incorporation

In addition to the promise of autonomy and freedom from regulatory oversight, there were financial incentives to incorporating the IM center. The PC structure would provide the means to increase revenues and corporate salaries. Senior administrators were trying to show that their model was going to work in an outpatient clinical setting. They believed strongly that the outpatient clinical practice would not only be successful enough to cover its own cost but would spin off profit that would support the teaching and research components, which would otherwise not be profitable.

They wanted to create incentives for the physicians to grow the practice by linking bonuses to patient volume—in the hospital setting, that is not possible. Under the PC structure, the center would

---

[2] The Stark regulations provide exceptions for institutions affiliated with a medical school, university, or government entity.

not be constrained by the hospital's human resources policy about base salaries. The market demand was high for the kind of providers they wanted to recruit, which pushed salaries above the HR base salaries for the hospital. If they couldn't pay these higher salaries, they would not be able to recruit for the center.

The assumption that the IM center would be extremely lucrative was a primary impetus to incorporate it as a separate entity yet keep it within the administrative structure of the existing foundation.

> They expected that within a year, this thing would be minting money. [IM Provider P11]

Once the IM center was approved by the board, the foundation advanced a seed fund to set up a scaled-down clinic and funds for a center resident and fellow. In partnership with a local research organization, the center also received a grant that helped offset salary costs for the director and two more fellows. However, the initial seed-fund loan was also slated to help pay for credentialing CAM providers, start-up legal costs, and salaries for the executive-level PC owners.

Forming a PC proved to be exceedingly complex. The center had advance funding from the board to set it up, but many of the people involved worked in the hospital. For the legal and administrative services it received from the hospital, the PC needed a contract to pay for staff time. The hospital also had contracts with the PC to pay for resident education and for a fellowship in integrative medicine. And the center paid for some time its own director spent overseeing the allied health professionals and acupuncturists, writing, and coming to meetings. The existence of many different contracts led to more complexity.

The center was structured as a PC under the hospital foundation but legally distanced from the hospital. The original plan was to have the center provide CAM services on a cash-only outpatient basis, to avoid third-party payment billing and reimbursement issues. However, because the PC was under the umbrella of the medical system (i.e., the foundation), the center was subject to hospital-wide policies. As a result, the center was required to hire the hospital's billing department to handle its accounts and to accept both public and private health insurance.

So, although the PC was conceived as a cash-only practice, because of its relationship with the hospital, it had to accept a mix of public and private third-party payments.

> The original model that [was] proposed was the model after [a local high-end clinic]. It's a cash-on-the-barrel model—no insurances. [They] sell herbs and homeopathic products and everything else out of the office, which we weren't going to do, but it was going to be cash on the barrel. And then our CFO said, "Oh, no, you can't do that because hospital employees may want to use the services there, so you have to take Blue Cross and Prudent Buyer." I said, "Okay, we'll take Blue Cross and Prudent Buyer." [Administrator P6]

Marketing the Center

To ensure its viability, the center needed a coordinated and sustained marketing and public relations campaign. However, perhaps because people assumed that the hospital's prestigious reputation would make such a campaign unnecessary, no funding was set aside for this purpose.

Marketing Context

External factors strongly influenced the marketing efforts of the center's administrators. Managed care has resulted in substantial increases in power among third-party payers, creating difficulty for broad marketing of CAM modalities that are not covered by these insurers. But while third-party payers may have constrained CAM use among segments of the population, television and the Internet have contributed to increased patient awareness of CAM and other medical options, including, increasingly, pharmaceuticals. The corollary to medicine as a business enterprise, in which patients are the consumers, is patients as savvy customers who expect to be able to choose among an array of medical options.

You need the intellectual and the academic integrity and collegial networking so that you become a known entity within the [CAM] world. People are on the Internet, they're reading books, they're looking at lectures, they're reading journals, and they are getting name identifications. I'll go with Weil, for example. Nobody in the country doesn't know [him]. Nobody in the country doesn't know Deepak Chopra. That wasn't by accident. That was by design. He's a brilliant marketer. That's kind of what it takes to make a success. [IM Provider P29]

The hospital's hierarchical structure promotes a particular culture, and an effective marketing campaign would have to explicitly address and negotiate these organizational features. As one informant said, this was an institution where everything was quid pro quo.

Branding Integrative Medicine

The integrative medicine center was established to capture an unmet niche market: patients who were seeking CAM care in a hospital environment and those who were open to or preferred a physician trained in both biomedicine and some modality of CAM. Given the center's location—near a proliferation of both high- and low-end CAM providers—the PC owners hoped to capture substantial market share for this untapped medical niche. The center director hired CAM providers to meet the perceived preferences of the local community.

We are two to three miles away from X. There are all kinds of practitioners out there. There are practitioners in Y who do nothing but CAM. So from a marketing point of view, there would really be nothing particularly unique [about providing a single CAM modality] . . . . We didn't think our role in the community was to replicate alternative complementary medicines that were in the community already. We didn't understand what value we would be bringing to the community just by doing that . . . that doesn't seem to be meeting a community need out there. But the blending of the two we thought would be valuable. [Administrator P12]

Why [we] picked those models, those kind of therapies, it was that those supposedly were the easiest to integrate. If you looked at utilization data that was available at the time, especially Eisenberg's articles, those are the services that patients were asking for. And then it would also capitalize on some of the ethnic particularities of our city. In other words, if you were in Dubuque, Iowa, maybe people wouldn't know what an acupuncturist was so much. But here we have such a large Asian population that it's not such a hard sell. So those were the services [we] picked first . . . acupuncture, chiropractic, traditional Chinese medicine, which could include more than acupuncture . . . that's licensed. [IM Provider P2]

External Marketing

The IM center's external marketing made use of biomedical and CAM professionals and the population surrounding the center. The director drew on the traditional means of marketing a practice or research: meet and greet, the lecture circuit, and education were prominent aspects of the effort. Numerous respondents noted that the director was an effective lecturer and was successful in marketing the IM center.

[The director] is a very effective speaker. I heard [the director] speak once at [a local] country club, and the audience was in the palm of [the director's] hand. [Board P14]

Internal Marketing

Because the center hoped to develop a referral network within the hospital, most of the marketing efforts focused on raising the visibility of the new center among hospital staff. The center staged noon conferences to evaluate supplements that would be known to most of the audience, reviewing the evidence for the supplements' use, common uses and effects, and possible drug interactions, among other things. The center also used grand rounds—the traditional means of disseminating information and research findings in a hospital.

When [the director] talked at the recent rounds to OB/GYN about what could be done for breech birth to turn the baby around through alternative therapies, you could see every person in that room listening. Because that's important. Who wants to be in a hospital for five days because of complications from a breech birth? And who wants a C-section? . . . [The director's] work, particularly on the educational front, is very instrumental in changing people's perceptions that it's not necessarily acupuncture, it's not actually visualization. There are therapeutic remedies that can be brought to bear to assist in the treatment of certain ailments and illnesses. I've been to lectures that [have been given] to overflow audiences . . . . [Expert P10]

Anticipating that the greatest obstacle to the center's success would be physician resistance, the center used these presentations as a means of dampening resistance. They also drew on an "insider"—the first integrative medicine fellow—to meet and greet physicians one-on-one to address their concerns and generate referrals. The IM fellow knew a lot of the medical staff because he had served three years as a resident and a fourth year as chief resident. He knew which doctors would be interested in CAM.

The center also attempted to improve its visibility by marketing to potential financial donors, providing pro bono continuing medical education (CME) lectures, and distributing flyers to hospital staff. The center administrators already knew from their own information that many hospital employees were using CAM.

Research and Training Efforts

While the center's training and research components were eclipsed by its emphasis on clinical care, they were part of the initial business plan. In fact, the training efforts began even before the center opened. Research efforts grew over time, particularly as the center began to accrue substantial debt and the additional revenue from research funds was increasingly needed to offset low reimbursement. In one project, a cardiothoracic surgery group investigated the use of acupuncture, massage, and guided imagery in the management of postoperative pain after coronary artery bypass grafting. Several other multidisciplinary studies were planned but never funded. The center director landed a research grant with an outside organization that accounted for the bulk of the center's research efforts. The IM center's two fellows were also involved with this research work.

From a broader socioeconomic perspective, it is important to note that the IM center was established during an overall funding downturn for academic research. Hospitals across the United States have been facing deficits and closures. Even with its stellar reputation, the hospital was facing financial constraints, including a low census and space limitations.

> It seems to me that academic medical centers in general have problems. If you've read any of the [local medical school's] reports in the last couple of months about how about a month ago they only had $20,000 in cash on any given day for floating their stuff there. Clearly [the others] are having similar types of difficulties, or maybe even more. I don't know if they're unique to [the hospital], but I will tell you that a number of my faculty come from other places. Some of them came from Pennsylvania, some of them came from Alabama, some of them came from Duke, Johns Hopkins, whatever. It does seem to be an issue across the board but nothing as big as what we see here. [Administrator P70]

Unlike many academic medical centers, this hospital's primary focus is clinical care rather than teaching or research, which made the fit of an IM model in this private hospital setting more problematic. However, a lot of research was going on for a nonuniversity private hospital.

For example, in comparing a neighboring university hospital, a board member elaborates on the difference in the case study hospital's focus on inpatient clinical care in contrast to traditional medical schools where the hospital, in effect, supports medical training.

> One of the key differences is that they are fundamentally a medical school running a hospital to accommodate the medical school.

We are fundamentally a hospital with research and teaching to support our fundamental mission, which is the hospital. [Board P22]

Yet, the mission of the hospital is to serve research and teaching, in addition to its clinical focus. The IM center met these needs by incorporating each of these core values in its model.

The Model and Research

Other hospital programs previously led successful research efforts that the center hoped to piggyback on or emulate. The center model that was implemented highlighted its research and teaching components, but implementing these components was difficult.

And there was going to be a three-part program. We were going to have a clinical arm which was going to be one big laboratory. And we were going to hire MDs who would integrate some of the therapies into their practice and would look at some of the common problems such as hypertension, diabetes, [and] asthma, and compare outcomes using previously established research programs designed to measure outcomes for drug studies . . . use those tools to look at outcomes and compare it to standard therapy. A second area was going to be research, the black box type of research, to see if the integrative medicine approach was better than traditional medicine, and then—if it was—to try to break down what the components were. But [there was] also the more traditional drug-type research, looking at herbs and other therapies for different illnesses. And then there was going to be a big teaching component, teaching for our house staff, our attending staff, and the public. That was how we were going to set it up. [Administrator P6]

Internal Academic Appointments

The hospital faculty underwent an internal review process for hospital appointment. Successful candidates interested in teaching were offered an additional appointment as an assistant professor at a local university that houses a medical school.

The faculty practice is kind of an IPA [Independent Practice Association] group unto itself, and they will bill for themselves, but they're still faculty. Whether they're 100 percent faculty or 50 percent faculty, I don't really know, but they're faculty. Somehow, part of their paycheck is related to them belonging to that university and teaching those residents. [We] have 150 obstetricians on staff, and I have a faculty of about 10. Out of the 150, about 8, maybe 10 teach the residents. [But] if they want to become part of the teaching program, they have to submit [an application] as anyone would for an academic affiliation. Our academic affiliations are the doctors here from [University X]. So my docs are affiliated and they're assistant professors and professors at [University X]. [Administrator P70]

Training

The center established a residency program, with comprehensive CAM training. This part of the program was judged by most commentators, including those who participated in it, to have gone well.

I had no direct experience in CAM, but everything that I was learning was through the acupuncture piece. Just the two of us; two brains are always better than one . . . [Training in herbs was also] part of the fellowship . . . we would, on a weekly basis, have a several-hour intensive course in herbal background, theory, and pharmacology. [IM Provider P11]

From an educational standpoint, I got an excellent education from [the director] on herbal medicine and on the integration of CAM with medicine, how it theoretically should work. I [also] had the opportunity to do the acupuncture course. [IM Provider P11]

Some of the training, particularly for acupuncture, occurred outside the institution.

The director and some staff members made sustained efforts to ensure that the in-house training component of the IM center was successful. In addition to the grand rounds, noon seminars, CME lectures, and other internal venues, the director led a weekly seminar.

> It was a once-a-week seminar that taught me about western European herbals and botanicals. We would meet with a very diverse group of physicians, pharmacists, and some alternative health [care] providers. We would each do research and talk about herbals and botanicals, choosing either a subject (like a disease) or a symptom (like abdominal pain or gastritis or migraines) and then talk about what we knew about all herbs in that category. Or we'd talk about one specific herb. We sort of switched off. Over a couple years we covered many, many herbs and many, many disease entities. It was a fabulous learning experience for me. [Hospital Provider P42]

External Training/Education Efforts
The education program also involved a large amount of activity outside the institution, such as giving presentations at both the local and national level. Because the center was an innovative program, it quickly gained a reputation in the IM community. The seminars were well-attended events.

> I participated in one talk that [the hospital] put on, where there must have been 500 people from the community who came. [Expert P37]

Research
The original research plan was to set up the center to collect outcomes data on patients. The educational arm of the center trained fellows in research and teaching skills. Some had previous training in health services research, and the center also began to prepare research proposals.

The director was able to secure funding for a study of CAM and hepatitis C. In addition, the director participated in research with a team outside the hospital that was awarded a large NCCAM grant. The director also began to develop research projects with local colleagues outside the center. But the research that eventually came about was not that which was conceived in the original plan.

Evidence-Based Practice and CAM/IM

Some respondents asserted that hard scientific evidence, such as that provided by randomized controlled trials (RCTs)—the gold standard of biomedicine—would be necessary to establish CAM's credibility in the biomedical community. Those who voiced this perspective stressed the issue of efficacy. From their vantage point, CAM needed to be tested and quantified.

> [CAM needs] the same standard of evidence that I need for clinical trials. Things that I use all the time. The best are the randomized controlled clinical trials. That's the standard that we hold ourselves to all the time. [Hospital Provider P87]

Physician perspectives about evidence-based medicine, however, were broad and included approaches that were more patient-centered. Some providers were willing to reduce the burden of proof for CAM. They were willing to accept quality of life outcomes over life expectancy for massage patients with end-stage cancer.

> I don't know anything about massage therapy. I can't really believe that it's anything other than having a wonderful placebo effect . . . maybe I'm just not familiar with the data. If someone told me that there is actually data to support the fact that people live three days longer with metastatic cancer if they got a massage, gosh, three extra days at the end of your life sounds good. If there was just some tangible proof. [Hospital Provider P88]

A minority of providers were reflective about biomedicine's limitations and flaws. These providers were aware that scientific results are often suppressed if they could have a negative impact on established paradigms or on a company's reputation or a product's marketability. They were also aware that when long-standing biomedical practices are subjected to the scrutiny of RCTs, the outcomes sometimes contradict decades of false assumptions and deleterious effects on patients' health. Respondents noted that as CAM practices are subjected to the rigors of scientific testing, some are meeting these criteria and then are adopted into biomedicine.

Some traditional physicians were open to using CAM without hard scientific evidence. They supported its use without such evidence either as a last resort or because they had experience with a particular CAM protocol to which their patients responded well.

> I've used it as an adjunct to less than satisfactory pain management overall. It's something I'm willing and happy to use, but it's out of desperation. It's not a fair analysis or opportunity for me to say how good it is. I trust it when I've read that it helps relieve [pain] sometimes, so I'm willing to accept that. It certainly isn't going to hurt. [Hospital Provider P87]

Some biomedical providers took a more pragmatic approach and frankly didn't care if there was scientific evidence to support CAM. They were open to it if it would help their patients.

> I don't have to know how it helps. I don't have to have the science. I really don't care. It's not what I'm interested in. But I need to know it's there and that it's available and that there are people who are experts in it who can see the patient. It would have been useful to refer patients there. [Hospital Provider P38]

Yet others made it clear that, to be accepted by the establishment, CAM must legitimize itself using the same research methods for evidence that are used by the dominant institution, biomedicine.

The IM center was forged, in part, to address this issue by generating evidence-based research on CAM. The director was dedicated to broadening CAM's evidence base and was planning to conduct prospective studies.

> Our mandate from the beginning was to explore, through an affiliation with [the hospital], using their staff resources whenever and wherever possible, the benefits of integrative medicine,

and, specifically, original research into botanicals to create new herbal products that would overcome the prejudices of the medical establishment by being patented and proven by clinical trials: first in vivo, second in vitro, third with human clinical subjects. [Expert P10]

The center wanted to avoid Food and Drug Administration (FDA) politics by not engaging in research that had anything to do with cancer, AIDS, or infectious diseases, and to limit its research to over-the-counter remedies. The purpose was to increase public awareness that natural medicine may be very effective and safe, as well as cost-effective.

Some biomedical providers noted that an evidence-based approach to CAM would provide an effective marketing tool. The need for evidence was also considered to be related to third-party payers for services—to provide evidence to gain reimbursements for CAM.

They don't reimburse any herbal supplements. Let's say that it does work and it would actually be cheaper. But it's difficult to get the study to prove that it works and, second, you can't get it reimbursed because there's no proof. So you see that catch-22? [Administrator P64]

Many of those interviewed stressed the importance of establishing evidence-based data for CAM to assuage safety concerns.

It's either effective or it's not effective. That's very nice. However, I would settle for a body of evidence that it's safe to take, that it doesn't have a drug interaction with the things I'm interested in it not interacting with, and that it has some either hypothetical or experiential benefit to treat the diseases I'm interested in treating. [Hospital Provider P88]

Competition and Referrals

The hospital's organizational structure fuels competition between its two cadres of providers: salaried faculty and freelancing private attending physicians. The IM center, therefore, entered a very competitive environment. And competition came from outside, too, as the center was established in an area that had a multitude of CAM providers and biomedical institutions.

External Competition

The IM center faced stiff competition from myriad small private practices and minor competition from local medical centers. The private practices included high-cost providers that catered to celebrities and depended on them to increase their market share. A host of CAM businesses operated in the city, including a wide range of small, low-cost providers in the nearby predominantly East Asian neighborhood. In addition, the hospital is bordered on the north, west, and south by competing medical centers. Finally, other hospital-based providers also offered CAM services. Patients who had previous positive experiences with any of these other providers might have been disinclined to seek care from the center's CAM providers.

> The problem was that a lot of patients who might come to see the doctor already have an outside acupuncturist. That became very difficult, because we would want them to work with the acupuncturist and they would say, "No." So they were really coming to see us as private physicians, but that doesn't build the whole center. [IM Provider P2]

> There wasn't a lot of integrative medicine actively happening inside the walls of [the hospital]. But clearly, around the periphery, a lot of private practice type stuff, a couple of the private attendings who work in the towers, the medical office buildings attached to the hospital, two EMT guys got in a traditional Chinese medicine practitioner and a chiropractor. In our catchment area there are just a lot of alternative medicine practitioners, independent freestanding solo practitioners. [IM Provider P3]

To understand the referral process among CAM and IM providers, and to determine whether CAM providers in the catchment area had any knowledge of the IM center's existence, we conducted face-to-face interviews with a snowball sample of 41 CAM providers. Table 4.1 describes the distribution of CAM modalities in this sample.

Awareness of the Center

Sixty percent of the CAM providers in this group had heard something about the IM center; however, most had only cursory knowledge about the services the center provided. Some were aware of its research component; a handful knew about the center through its director.

About half the CAM providers who had heard of the center had negative opinions about it, ranging from complaints about large hospital settings and politics to logistical issues such as parking problems and the lack of IM center providers' availability.

> It's a huge organization. What I know is there are the politics and now the organization of this. Parking is a terrible thing. The environment has to be much more friendly, like any outpatient clinic has to be much more friendly. [CAM Provider P1]

Table 4.1
Distribution of CAM Provider Modalities

CAM Modality	n
Doctor of Chiropractic	7
Integrative Medicine Doctor	6
Licensed Acupuncturist	7
Naturopath/Herbalist	5
Massage Therapist	7
Other	5
Homeopathic (not MD)	4

Half of the CAM providers said they would need more information about the center before making any referrals.

> I would actually have to know more about what the center does. But right now, I'd never refer anyone there, because I don't know what they do. [CAM Provider P20]

Referral Process

While a few providers believed that the "pie was big enough to share," more were threatened by potential competition from the IM center and, consequently, would not refer patients there. Further, respondents reported that they thought the center was providing services that established CAM practitioners were already providing.

> I don't feel it's as accessible to a practitioner like me. I mean, that's a place where, if I sent a patient, I might expect to never see them again. [CAM Provider P4]

> The kind of work they were doing was duplicating what I do in conjunction with the referral base that I have. So, for instance, if I were seeing someone who I felt needed western medication for pain or some other intervention like biofeedback, I have my own sources for all that. [CAM Provider P2]

Other providers attempted to build relationships with the center but encountered availability issues.

> I was asked to contact someone there, and he and I played phone tag for a while. I never pursued it anymore because I felt like I didn't get a lot of feedback. So I don't know a whole lot. [CAM Provider P5]

Many of the external CAM providers were wary of potential competition from an IM center and made disparaging comments about large hospitals. However, they wanted to hear more about the center and its model, and seemed open to possible future connection with it if more information were available to them about the providers and the modalities offered.

> If I knew the doctors who worked there and if they have a good reputation . . . . I would like to know what they do, then, yes, of course I would refer patients to the IM center. [CAM Provider P10]

The CAM providers' referral process consisted of a decisionmaking tree motivated by push-and-pull mechanisms and hindered by obstacles. Figure 4.2 illustrates these driving forces.

In summary, the perceptions that outside CAM providers had about the IM center, their lack of knowledge about it, and the obstacles identified in the referral process conspired against the center's receiving patient referrals from local CAM providers. Essentially, no viable network was established with these stakeholders.

Figure 4.2
CAM Providers Referral Process

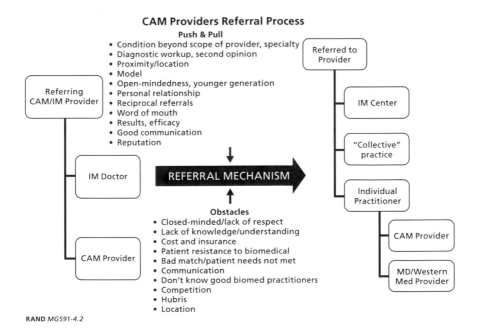

RAND MG591-4.2

Internal Competition

Like most academic medical settings, the hospital, with its fairly rigid internal hierarchies, fosters internal competition among staff, including among types of providers. Competition is particularly marked between the full-time faculty (who ostensibly earn a certain salary regardless of patient volume because they also teach, although that appears to have changed in the present medical economic climate) and the private practice attending physicians (who generate their own income and generate a profit for the hospital). A third group of providers, who are hired on contract (e.g., emergency care) and practice at a distance from the internal hospital hierarchies, appear to be less affected by turf issues.

> At [the hospital], when a new program starts, they want to be very careful not to take business away from the attending physicians. [The hospital] has people who are on staff. They have 800 people in the community who have privileges [to admit patients]. They are a powerful lobby. When anything new at [the hospital] is starting, there's a lot of concern about not taking patients away from those doctors. Their income and their livelihood are tied to how many patients they see. [IMM Provider P17]

The salaried faculty generally prefer to keep CAM treatments in-house, providing them in their own departments; however, their fear of the IM center as competition was potentially manageable through building reciprocal referral paths and collaborating on grants. Of the two groups, the private attending physicians had the most to lose by referring their patients to an IM center run by an internist with other internists and a doctor of osteopathic medicine (DO) on staff. The attending physicians might fear that the center would "steal" their patients.

Not all providers saw the center as competition. Some saw it as providing care that drew on a different market or providing services that were different enough from the care they provided to be non-threatening. Other providers noted that the center was not a threat to them, because they offered these services themselves and, therefore, would not refer patients to the IM center.

I use it [a particular combination of herbs] on a lot of patients. But I've got experience with it, and I would prescribe that myself. [Hospital Provider P81]

Fear of competition had never prevented the hospital from instituting something new.

The IM Center in Operation: A Profile

Personnel and Staffing
At the peak of the center's operations, the staff consisted of the integrative MD director, a fellow MD trained in acupuncture who gained junior attending status several months after the clinic opened, another fellow MD, an osteopath, two part-time acupuncturists, a part-time massage therapist, a nurse, and an administrator. The front desk reception phones were answered by a call service located elsewhere, and billing was contracted out to the main hospital.

Physical Description of the Center
The center consisted of a rented suite of three exam rooms in a building adjacent to the hospital complex. According to accounts from administrators, providers, and patients, the space was inadequate to accommodate the providers or all the patients.

You had conflicts with provider schedules; you had limited room as far as how many exam rooms we have to see patients. We at times had to borrow exam rooms because there was just not enough space that we had allocated when providers were together to see all the patients. [Administrator P20]

Providers worked in cramped quarters and had to convert exam rooms into offices. There was no private consultation space—staff could use the conference room if it was available. The lack of space meant that the center could not expand and accommodate more patients.

The décor and ambience were clinical and sterile, according to the providers who worked there. The sense of integration in terms of the physical space was nonexistent.

> The ambience, the environment of the place was so clinical and obviously, yes, you are in a hospital. But this was supposed to be a place for people to come to forget that they were going through chemotherapy treatment. Or to forget that they had horrible bouts of IBS or they had horrible pain. I learned about color therapy and music therapy and all these wonderful things that we should have been using. Instead we were just given this tiny little place with these three little offices, and sterile everything. [IM Provider P50]

In the IM paradigm, spatial layout is an important issue.

> From a feng shui point of view, it's wrong. I think you need to play music. You need candlelight. You need so many things to make it really integrative. We still were operating in a very western clinical environment, where everything was very medical and sterile, and it wasn't integrative to my taste. That's my feeling about it. [IM Provider P24]

Space issues also affected the ability to train and teach. By the second year, virtually no medical students came through the center, although many asked to do so. Training was impossible because the clinic was so small there was no room for additional bodies.

IM Center Patients

The patients were major stakeholders, so it is important to consider their opinions of the center and of CAM in general.

Patient Sample

We conducted telephone interviews with a random sample (n=40) of all patients (n=1,146) referred to the center over a three-year period (see Table 4.2). To capture potential differences across illness types, we stratified the

Table 4.2
IM Center Patient Sample, n=40

	High user (≥ 7 visits)	Low user (1–6 visits)	Total
Cancer	4	4	8
Pain	5	5	10
Symptoms/Conditions	7	7	14
General health/checkups	4	4	8
Total	20	20	40

sample by presenting problem and high or low service utilization. We used a random number generator with SAS software to select patients to contact. As in national data on CAM use, these patients were predominantly white (85 percent), female (85 percent), and 40–60 years old.

Health Care Choices

Why Patients Seek CAM/IM

Our findings were similar to those of other studies published in the United States, the United Kingdom, and Australia. Patients sought CAM to avoid the use of pharmaceutical drugs or because they felt that conventional biomedical treatment had a limited effect on their health problems. These concerns appeared to have contributed to their dissatisfaction with traditional biomedical care.

> I had breast cancer and a stroke and I was in my late 60s. I felt like I was going downhill. My primary care doctor kept saying, "But you're healthy," and I kept saying, "But I don't *feel* good." I started going to a community meeting that I saw in the paper about alternative health care and at one of them I just raised my hand and said, "Does anyone know of a medical doctor who does integrative medicine?" [IM Patient P14]

Most patients referred themselves to the center. The majority of these proactive patients wanted a biomedical physician with an integrative approach—somebody who combined a western and eastern approach to medicine; others reported that they had an affinity for homeopathy or preferred a "natural" approach.

Many patients learned about the center through their social networks of friends, family, and acquaintances. Some patients sought referrals within CAM-based social networks, such as health food stores, alternative community directories, vitamin manufacturers, or well-known CAM gurus on the book-selling and lecture circuit. Other patients heard about the center from the in-house lecture series and internal exchange systems, or were referred by staff physicians.

Why Patients Chose This Hospital for CAM Care

Few patients mentioned the reputation of the hospital, which is considerable, as the reason they sought care in this particular center. Instead, it was the reputation of the center director or the IM model of care that attracted them.

> I didn't choose [the hospital]. I chose [Dr. X] because I wanted a medical doctor. I didn't want to just go to a naturopath or something. I wanted a medical doctor who could do the things that were different than my primary care doctor could do. [IM Patient P14]

Some patients wanted to broaden their health care by being able to incorporate both biomedical and CAM approaches, recognizing that each has limitations. For others, an IM environment provided a biomedical safety net; in other words, the IM model made CAM care "quackproof."

> I wanted to try alternative methods, but I wanted an MD as well, somebody who would have knowledge of both. That was very, very important to me because I did not want to go off with somebody on an alternative path who—I don't want to say quack—but who might not be very well grounded in traditional medicine. I wanted somebody who knew both sides of the coin, who could

suggest alternatives to me but . . . also had the western medical background, which is important to me because I grew up with it. So using that as sort of the backdrop while then exploring the unknown other side. [IM Patient P17]

Convenience and access were not critical factors in patients' decision to go to the center. However, previous treatment at the hospital was a significant contributing factor; either because they were "comfortable" with the hospital or because they had established long-term relationships with various staff physicians. One respondent was born at the hospital.

Presenting Problems

Chronic conditions—often multiple chronic conditions, such as fibromyalgia or migraines—were the primary reasons that patients visited the center. Few patients initially entered the IM center because of an acute illness episode, although some came to the center for postoperative care. The majority of the patients were seeking care for multiple health concerns or for health maintenance.

I had a ruptured disc and had surgery. I've been in pain ever since. It flared up all other kinds of problems. I had fibromyalgia, irritable bowel syndrome—you name it—shingles at the end. [IM Patient P9]

We actually wanted to begin a relationship with a doctor there as far as getting a physical and just general health maintenance. That was what took us there, from the perspective of just having an ongoing health maintenance program. [IM Patient P31]

Patient Integration

About half the time, patients who saw a CAM/IM provider were also seeing a strictly biomedical caregiver. Overall, the key factor in whether patients decided to see a CAM or western biomedical provider was how they categorized their condition; that is, its severity and intractability. They tended to seek western medicine for serious or severe conditions or illnesses and mechanistic care (e.g., surgery)—what one patient called "fender work" or "nuts and bolts" health care needs. If their condition did not respond to those kinds of care, its persistence increased the odds that the patient would cross over to another medical model.

> [Making a decision about the type of provider to see] is complicated. It depends on the problem, who's available and what I feel like doing, and who I think will handle it best. Then other times, I will go to three people if the problem still continues. [IM Patient P35]

Biomedicine and the Hospital Environment

The majority of the patients preferred providers who were physicians with training in western medicine but, as medical consumers, they wanted more choices than western medicine offers. The patients in our hospital-based sample also cited the efficacy and appropriateness of western medicine, particularly if they had significant health problems or needed to "be put back together again."

> They provided me with a knowledge about things I knew nothing about that I wanted to know more about. I wanted someone who was also a medical doctor because of my extensive health issues. I'm on a lot of drugs. I have thyroid problems; I have high blood pressure. [Dr. X] has me on red yeast rice to lower my cholesterol as opposed to Prylosec, which I love. She'll always give me options. [IM Patient P1]

Patients also felt that the biomedical approach provided a frame of credibility and increased their sense of comfort and safety.

> It was a comfort level from having grown up with western medicine. So I used that as a sort of backdrop while exploring the unknown on the other side. [IM Patient P17]

In addition, some patients believed that the biomedical and CAM interface was critical, either because of the seriousness of their condition or as a practical means of integrating their care across various providers.

Summary

The clinic was established as a for-profit outpatient clinic. It was administratively housed in a foundation but was a separate professional corporation. This PC was created to shield the center from the Stark regulations that prevented the hospital from owning such a clinic. However, the use of a PC was also partly dictated by the expectation that the center would be profitable and this structure would encourage the IM providers to see more patients and earn more money for themselves and the center.

No formal marketing plan was constructed. Within the hospital, the main marketing strategy was through educational programs (lectures and grand rounds). Externally, the clinic was constrained by the lack of a marketing budget and by hospital restrictions on where and how it could market itself. The main method of marketing was presentations to local groups.

In the original plan, the center included a CAM research component that would conduct health services research on outcomes as well as research on herbal products. This did not happen, although the center did become involved in research projects with other units and with an outside organization.

Although IM providers did not receive academic appointments, the center was involved in considerable academic activity. It established a residency program with comprehensive CAM training, and staff participated in extension lectures, presentations, and rounds. The center was not able to develop a referral base among the local CAM community. Its referrals came from within the hospital, and they were limited.

At its peak, the IM center staff consisted of the MD director, a fellow MD trained in acupuncture who gained junior attending status several months after the clinic opened, another fellow MD, an osteopath, two part-time acupuncturists, a part-time massage therapist, a nurse, and an administrator. The problem of credentialing the CAM providers limited who could be employed. The clinic was housed next door to the hospital in a modest setting that had inadequate space for its services.

The patients who visited the IM center resembled those in the general literature on CAM use. They sought CAM to avoid the use of pharmaceutical drugs or because they thought conventional biomedical treatment had had a limited effect on their health problems. Chronic conditions, often multiple chronic conditions, were the primary reasons patients visited the center. Most were drawn to the center by the reputation of the director and/or the IM model of care.

CHAPTER FIVE

The Demise of the Center

Two years into the center's existence, the financial losses were such that the hospital administration began the process of shutting down the center and the corporation. The program was restructured within the Department of Medicine in 2001 and ceased to exist as an independent center at that time.

Financial Mission: "Stop the Bleeding"

Despite the board's insistence that loss-leader programs can be supported if they meet a perceived community need, programs that fail to contribute to overhead are more likely to be eliminated, especially given the hospital's current financial shortfall. In 2000, the first step in attempting to turn the center around financially was to piece together its initial business model and financial expectations. Two finance and management specialists were mandated to stem the center's future financial losses and reduce the previous year's deficit.

> This thing is bleeding to death, which at the end of the day impacts the entire organization. Get the bleeding down to [X amount of money]. It's still a for-profit corporation, but find a way to realign what's happening here with the expenses and the revenue, and only have it lose X dollars. [Even in] a not-for-profit organization, you have to make money. In not-for-profit, you take that profit and you put it back into the organization and you buy capital equipment, you do renovations, you do whatever. In a for-

profit corporation, first they pay the shareholders, then they take what's left and roll it back in. This is about either making it lose less or killing it. [Administrator P39]

The first goal was to streamline the center's structure by reducing its costs while keeping it in the same location. The hospital administration reduced the center's rent and the number of staff and providers, and the center attempted to increase its patient volume. However, a paper-based reduction of losses was insufficient. In fact, this approach may have been particularly unacceptable, as these losses would have to be "eaten." The board directive to the administration was to get the deficit down to a set dollar amount, and they did achieve that target. But the institution overall was not hitting its financial targets, so the board decided to cut programs that were not breaking even.

Some center staff members considered management's financial goals to be unrealistic, because the requirement for increased patient volume did not include necessary increases in space. The staff also believed that the center was not given enough time to produce a profit—they improved their numbers in the six months they were given, but the center was still closed.

At this point, the shortcomings of the center became obvious.

We were basically looking at the model to see what was wrong and why it wasn't working. Essentially, the numbers just didn't add up. It was set up with high-priced labor. Labor was much higher than you could afford, than reimbursement would handle. The environment that it was set up in was not really that conducive to this type of product. And it just didn't have the volume to support the overhead and the expenses eventually. The decision was made six months later just to close it down, because we just weren't making it. And it would never work. It would never work here at [the hospital], is the bottom line, in that current model. [Administrator P32]

So despite the changes, the outlook was grim for the center.

It's pretty clear [that] this is never going to make any money. It's always going to need to be supported. And then you start to look at how much effort you put into this pipsqueaky little program. How much time is it taking compared to cardiovascular surgery, which yields a contribution to overhead of millions? [Administrator P39]

The recommendation from the hospital administrators was to close down the corporation.

There's no joy in killing. You probably lose more money than people would in a real business, because we spend an awful lot of time trying to figure out how to save it. This thing should have probably been killed far earlier on, and we lost a lot more money because of a well-intended good effort. [Administrator P39]

Restructure

In 2001, the program was severely scaled back and restructured in the Department of Medicine, which suggests a question about the development and implementation of the center's business plan. Why was it now possible to see IM patients within the hospital's Department of Medicine?

It's a mothballed program, basically. It's still kind of operating. People go visit the battleship. They're walking around it and seeing all the things it used to be, but it's a shell of what it was. [Administrator P52]

Reactions to the "Kill"

The board was disappointed but accepted the decision to close the PC and restructure the center. In some cases, however, members were denying the reality, that "restructuring" was in many ways a euphemism for permanently mothballing the failed enterprise.

I felt like an advocate, but I wasn't a strong, active one. Many of us were. In fact, when it was cut back, there was a little groan around the room. I think the board was very hopeful that this was going to be successful, and, really, the whole plan was to go into it with a lot of optimism, so it was a disappointment that it didn't work, but we understood. There were some members who felt it was a bad idea to close it down and wanted that not to be a final decision. [Board P22]

Some of the hospital staff believed that the center had exceeded expectations because the implementation process involved certifying and securing hospital-wide privileges for the center's staff, which contributed to a significant cultural change in the hospital's attitude toward CAM. The center changed the perception of the medical staff and the mindset of some providers: Before the center's creation, no CAM providers were employed at the hospital; afterward, CAM providers were privileged as allied health professional staff, and they are now formally acknowledged by the MEC and the board.

Contributing Factors to Closure

The internal factors contributing to the decision to shut down the corporation included a perceived lack of resistance to the center's closure among hospital staff. As the hospital faced shrinking margins, programs that were costing money were recognized as a double handicap in terms of space and financial resources.

As a PC, the center was unable to use cost-shifting to absorb or buffer its losses. These losses could have been anticipated, as most hospital-based IM centers have not been big moneymakers; but the original task force seems to have overlooked the financial shortfalls of the IM programs it visited, focusing instead on studies documenting high rates of CAM use (which they failed to realize were not, for the most part, provider-mediated). There was a belated recognition that most hospital-based IM programs are not making money.

I went to a conference in Hawaii run by Eisenberg two years ago, specifically on setting up integrative medicine centers. Ninety percent of all these medical centers were not making any money. I think it's very hard with insurance today to accept all insurances with big companies doing the billing who maybe don't know the specifics of the billing. [Hospital Provider P42]

Also, the systemic problem of integrating a cash-only clinical model into an existing medical system's mixed-payer reimbursement structure was not unique to this IM clinic. Providers who order an MRI for headaches can get insurance reimbursement, but if a CAM provider offers manipulation for headaches, there will be no reimbursement. So accepting insurance is problematic with current billing codes, which makes the integrative approach systematically problematic.

The administration hurt the center by trying to make it a cash-only venture. Patients on Medicare were not willing or able to pay cash. If a service such as massage is available in physical therapy and is covered by Medicare, why would patients come to the center and pay for it themselves?

These broader problems were compounded by the hospital's planned expansion into a new building, which meant that it needed space. One solution was to free up space by eliminating programs that were not financially productive. Without a groundswell of support from the medical staff or a large consumer demand, the center didn't get much support in this climate of change.

The inadequate space allocated to the center further jeopardized its viability, and the hospital environment detracted from its potential for success because of inflexible system-wide policies and bureaucratic structure.

> The environment, as far as the setting itself, was small, it was crowded, it was an afterthought. It didn't have enough room. It wasn't private. It really isn't conducive, in my mind, to having a physical site to do integrative medicine. [Administrator P32]

There was also an increased fear of litigation for the IM center and a perceived need for increased vigilance and risk management because it was providing nonbiomedically based health care. The institution wanted MD oversight at the center, which was impractical and greatly increased costs.

Summary

The key factors that contributed to the center's demise and restructuring were financial, location, market share, image, normative patient expectations, and medical, as well as broader culture mores. The center was housed in an area adjacent to neighborhoods with high rates of both low- and high-end competition, which led one interviewee to speculate that it "lacked the guns" to compete. However, the problem of stiff competition is not unique to this IM center; it is a risk for any medical start-up that lacks the ability to acquire or merge with a lucrative established enterprise.

> But maybe one of the messages is that all health care, like all politics, is local. By way of example, we one time had a fairly significant program in reproductive medicine going on here. Our relationship with that individual was discontinued. We have not had any significant reproductive medicine program here since. And the main reason is, it's exactly the same circumstances. This is a business in this community that, if you wanted to start from scratch, you couldn't do it. There's too much competition. If the reports one hears from other settings, that integrative medicine gets killed because of an internal conspiracy, that's not the case here at all. Not in the least. If you were to ask me the one thing that caused the failure, I would say . . . stiff . . . competition. [Administrator P27]

In addition to its problematic location and the competition, the center had image problems. CAM clinics traditionally promote health and wellness, while hospitals are associated with disease and illness, so the hospital association was a detriment in this sense. Locating the center in a small, unattractive space that lacked any CAM or spa-like ambiance also contributed to its failure.

Also, because it was not viewed as a winner, the program was less attractive to the hospital as a candidate for philanthropy.

> From a policy or philosophy standpoint, we don't try to use philanthropy to shore up otherwise failing enterprises. We use philanthropy to provide value added and enhancements, and take

something that could do okay and make it great. [Administrator P27]

The impact of the internal conflict about images and expectations also should be examined as possibly contributing to the center's failure. Could CAM fit into the institution's ethos of "leading the pack"? And, perhaps more important, is it possible to reconcile the image of a prestigious hospital with the promotion of nonconventional practitioners?

Our culture, if you listen to the ads that we have, is about integration, excellence, leading the pack. That's our tag line. It doesn't fit. It can have a subline: If you ever need any of these things, then we have this program you can go to. But it doesn't meet "leading the pack." [Administrator P39]

What is also clear in this case study is that the top levels of the hospital hierarchy and the administrators who created the IM program did not agree on its definition.

A very interesting point that I think is a key issue [is] that everyone has a different image of what this program is going to look like. Is it going to be doctors in suits with acupuncture needles? Is it going to be wild African tribesmen with briefcases?

Is it going to be chiropractors coming in from the chiropractic college, doing admissions in the hospital? There's lots of scenarios. Everyone's going to have to sit down and really lay their cards on the table as to what their expectations are. Getting everyone's images out on the table. [Administrator P36]

The clash of images illustrates the cultural tensions that may be implicit in the acculturation process of integrating CAM and biomedicine. It suggests the need for long-term support if an IM center is to eventually surmount these problems and succeed.

But despite the significant financial losses and the ultimate demise of the center, some people still see it as a venture that added to the institution.

I really think that we did a great job of planning, despite the outcome. I think we did a great job of getting board and administrative and medical staff understanding. We didn't rush it. Of course, it is different now than when we started doing this. It was more of a model for change, generally, rather than specifically about CAM. It was a good model. We took our time. We got the appropriate body and support. We did the scientific literature and the site visits. For a radical change, which was radical in an institution like that, I think that was an excellent process. I think we had a model that was appropriate for who and what we were. We weren't trying to be different than our mission and our character. It just turned out that there was no market for it, although we thought there was. We wanted to have a model by which the practice of medicine could be changed. And, conversely, the practice of CAM could be changed. We were essentially an alpha site for the concept of integrative practice. [Administrator P13]

CHAPTER SIX

Evaluation

In Chapter Three, we told the story of the planning for the integrative medicine center (IM center); in Chapter Four, we described the implementation and operation of the center; and in Chapter Five, we told of the center's ultimate closing. These chapters were intended to be primarily narrative and descriptive. In this chapter, we present an evaluative discussion of the results of our stakeholder analysis. We assess outcomes and the impact of the decisions and forces that shaped the center's creation, operations, and eventual demise. These results form the basis for our conclusions in Chapter Seven.

Legal Issues

Legal issues were responsible for shaping the center as a private corporation under the foundation.

The Decision to Incorporate
The Stark regulations (described in Chapter Three) presented serious impediments to establishing an IM center as part of a private hospital and provided motivation for creating the center as a professional corporation (PC). But the PC structure did more than circumvent the regulations against the corporate practice of medicine; it provided a strategic way to increase revenues and corporate salaries. From a risk-reduction vantage point, the PC eliminated hospital liability for CAM/IM services and for any financial losses. At the same time, it protected the center from Medical Executive Committee (MEC) oversight and

hospital-wide salary caps. The PC model also would allow the center to tie provider bonuses to patient volume. Finally, this physician-friendly corporation would have been able to offer stock options.

The center's creators anticipated that incorporating the IM center would provide regulatory shelter and support an entrepreneurial corporate structure to increase physician incentives, but it also brought extra costs, particularly for start-up. For example, the center could not take advantage of the hospital's preexisting salary structure and had to pay for items such as rented space, a billing service, and extra insurance.

> That's where a lot of our financial burden came in, because we had to replicate a lot of stuff that the hospital already had. [IM Provider P5]

Credentialing and Licensing

One of the center's legal successes was to design and implement policies and procedures for credentialing and garnering hospital privileges for CAM providers, a significant challenge in the administrative structure of the hospital's medical system. Given the importance of this issue, and because of the difficulties that arose, we discuss it separately. The administrators decided to use only licensed practitioners, which meant they had to address both state and local regulations.

State-level certification of CAM providers in California was a particularly difficult issue for the center's acupuncture care. While chiropractors are licensed at the state level, acupuncturists can be licensed nationally or at the state level. However, in California, acupuncturists must obtain a California state license, which requires a four-year master's degree in traditional Oriental medicine, even if they already have a national licensure.

In addition, local regulations affected the IM center's hiring of massage therapists. There is no national certification or educational requirement for massage; therapists register with the police department and acquire a business permit in the city in which they practice. The hospital is technically in city X but is adjacent to cities Y and Z, so IM center massage therapists often needed to acquire multiple city-specific permits.

The decision to employ only licensed CAM providers excluded some common CAM modalities, such as naturopathy, whose practitioners were not licensed in California until 2006 (although they were licensed in 17 other states). Thus, the center's hiring process was influenced by whether a provider had a license or permit. For example, one CAM provider was hired because he held dual licensure while other providers, with whom the director had worked and whom she respected, could not be hired because they lacked the necessary external credentials.

Internally, establishing a functioning IM center required the design and implementation of a credentialing process for allied health professionals. The center's developers implemented a program that established "rules, regulations, procedures, and policies" for credentialing CAM providers within the hospital. This seemed like a small matter, but it was a significant success of the IM center enterprise. The program has been adopted by other hospital centers; for example, by the cardiac center when it wanted to hire CAM providers.

> Before this happened, nobody on the [hospital] staff was a chiropractor, massage therapist, acupuncturist; it was not available. Today, it's available. [CAM providers are] on the allied health professional staff. They've formally been acknowledged by the Medical Executive Committee and the board [so] that these kinds of people can exist [within the hospital]. There's an approval process, an application process, and a privileging process . . . in place. [Administrator P13]

Business Plan

Along with the legal factors, the business plan (or lack thereof) had a tremendous impact on the center. From the very start, the business plan proved to be problematic. The plan's most significant—and perhaps fatal—flaw was that it was structured on faulty premises and assumptions.

> Within the first 18 months it was [assumed that the center was] going to be grossing a million and a half dollars. It just wasn't going to happen. [Provider P1]

The other assumption was that they would get an economic return on a visit. However, they did not realize how few patients they could run through the space that was available. The expectation that it would take less than two years to become very profitable was not realistic.

The task force used the following assumptions to create the business plan: high patient volume (based on reports of high levels of local CAM use); high levels of in-house referrals; strong revenues; a large population of CAM adherents willing to come to a hospital for their CAM care; and a single-payer client who would be willing and able to pay for visits with cash, regardless of potential insurance reimbursement. These false assumptions led the task force to conclude that a large local medical niche market existed and the hospital could tap into this parallel revenue stream.

The task force and the board may have misinterpreted the data about high rates of CAM use when they established the IM center. In particular, the majority of the CAM modalities in the 1993 Eisenberg, Kaptchuk, and Arcarese study were not provider-mediated (e.g., herbal supplements), meaning that an IM center would not profit from them.

> The data on the number of people using CAM and the amount spent on CAM is the biggest falsehood that has caused all of these people to make the wrong assumptions. All these money numbers come out, and everybody who's starting an integrative program has dollar signs in their eyes. That is the only reason that integrative medicine made its way into the hospitals. [IM Provider P11]

In the center's business plan, this misinterpretation was further compounded by the attempt to emulate an existing local model that catered to a single-payer population of entertainment industry elites and other wealthy clients. Moreover, the business plan assumed and expected that providers with this kind of patient base would refer patients to the newly formed IM center.

[They thought that] these very well-to-do doctors who are seeing hundreds of thousands of patients [would] send all their patients here. When they hospitalize their patients, they're going to send them to us. Then we'll get involved with them and start collaborating with them and do research. We'll form this big happy network of integrative medicine doctors, and we'll all sing "Kumbaya," and we'll make lots of money. That's a flawed approach to begin with. [Expert P37]

The developers failed to ground their plan with sound measures to ensure and grow a diversified patient and referral base either internally or externally. Internally, they did not conduct a hospital-wide needs assessment or coordinate efforts across departments to develop and nurture trust or to develop and sustain consistent referral patterns.

To be successful, such a program needs a patient or referral base. The developers should also have determined whether similar programs were making money and researched the payer mix and the services patients were paying for, as well as what they were spending. None of this was done.

I think the reason everybody thought alternative medicine was so attractive is it's a cash business. And the American public, based upon pretty good research, was spending a lot of money on alternative medicine, so we wanted to get in on that. Maybe that's the wrong reason to start a program. There was never an assessment of needs of each particular department or division. There weren't point people or representatives [who] would determine [the needs for specific modalities for specific departments]. [Hospital Provider P73]

Moreover, the fledgling program failed to secure the kind of long-term financial support necessary to build its reputation, referral system, and patient base. There was no long-term funding.

Rather than pursuing market research, the business plan assumed strong patient and provider referral bases and a single-payer client type that would meet the goals of maximizing five full-time employees (FTEs), including a director, two acupuncturists, a chiropractor, and a massage therapist. Further, the business model projected that the center would provide services to patients seven hours a day, six days a week. The creators assumed that it would function at 50 percent capacity during the first quarter, 80 percent by the fourth quarter, and 100 percent within the following 15 months. The financial projections assumed "fairly brisk growth in year 1 and continued levels of high productivity throughout years 2 and 3," with projected payments of 60 percent fee-for-service at 6 months, 75 percent at 12 months, 80 percent at 24 months, and 85 percent at 36 months. In year 2 it was assumed that the center would need to hire two additional part-time CAM providers to meet "increased patient volume." The reality was very different: There was an inverse arc in fee-for-service payments, a reduction in staff, and a steady decline in growth and capacity.

In addition to the unrealistic proposed growth pattern, the PC business plan overlooked the high start-up costs and ignored the need for long-term funding to build and sustain growth until the center reached profitability. Each of these flawed projections contributed to the center's failure to thrive. While the overhead in a large, well-established medical corporation might be able to absorb such a growing debt, the center's financial vulnerability was ensured when it was incorporated as a private entity without an overall vision or a realistic and detailed operating budget, or the ability to shift costs.

> If you try to start off paying full salaries for 100 percent productivity while you're ramping up, you're obviously not going to make it. And somebody has to fund that, whether you get donor dollars or whether the institution makes an institutional decision [to] fund this for X period of time, and then if these targets and these financial criteria [are not met], then the program is cut. [Administrator P65]

The center's independence as a PC hurt it and trapped it in a poor financial state. If it had been a department in the hospital, it could have used the hospital's infrastructure to help offset some expenses. If it had been set up as a regular department and affiliated with another department, such as physical rehabilitation, it could have shared some labor costs and economies of scale, and might have fared better.

Because of the center's novel approach to health care, it was critical that its business model be founded on clarity of vision outlined in a mission statement and supplemented by a detailed, workable operating budget. But instead of a sound business model, the program had what amounted to an approach of "build it and they will come." This attitude was noted by mid-level managers as the combined effects trickled down to the center's front line. From a management perspective, the center's business model lacked the basics to succeed: a detailed strategic plan and a viable operating budget. These basics needed to be codified and accessible, particularly to those running and working in the center. To the managers, it appeared that there was no strategic plan. Also, there was some doubt about the priority given to the center.

> If they want it to be more successful, then they're going to have to give it a higher priority and give it some resources, and rethink the business plan. [Hospital Provider P87]

A center within the Department of Medicine might have been able to conceal its losses, which could have been absorbed in the department's overhead costs long enough to enable it to become a viable, recognized entity. The independent center that was envisioned would draw from a broad patient base through a multihospital referral structure, with a robust payer mix, and would be held as a corporation by IM practitioners. This plan might have resulted in greater resilience over time with a broader revenue base and time to grow market share, develop marketable panache, and increase stakeholder stewardship. However, in reality, the center drew on a small patient base in a location with significant market competition.

Mission Statement

Adding to the difficulties was the lack of a mission statement for the model that was implemented. One early business plan outlined the following vision and goals:

- A world-class clinical program that integrates CAM therapies with primary care.

- A premier education component to train physicians and provide information to industry and third-party payers on CAM.
- A research program focusing on outcome, efficacy, and cost-effectiveness of CAM.
- A center of excellence as a prototype for future integrative centers.

When the first director was interviewed for the position, the center director was asked to produce a vision statement. The one he produced included medicine, research, and education. This was a very broad outline and was not used as an official document. Board members and administrators mentioned the importance of a mission statement as it applied to the hospital but not to the center itself. We were unable to uncover a final mission statement for the IM center.

Image, Location, and Market Share

In addition to the structural flaws of the business plan, four key factors contributed to the center's lack of profitability: image, location/market share, normative patient expectations, and medical and broader cultural mores.

First, the hospital-based center lacked the ambience of high-end CAM clinics, and it lacked adequate space. The patients were not enthusiastic about the center's setting and environment. They complained that it was "meager," "very boxy and institutional feeling . . . no windows," "old," and "kind of plain." But the most frequent complaint was that it was too small. The cramped space raised privacy problems by violating policies regarding patient confidentiality; it also disrupted patients' treatment experience.

Second, the hospital's location—near a predominantly East Asian neighborhood that offers low-cost CAM and surrounded by communities with a number of CAM providers—meant that it was operating in a saturated market.

Third, patients may have been unfamiliar with or resistant to the possibility of integrative care, with its one-stop shopping; they did not embrace this proposed niche market. For example, many patients who were satisfied with the center wanted a specific IM clinician to become their primary care physician, derailing the planned "consultant" referral model.

Fourth, CAM may have posed too much of a threat to the dominant medical mores. Tension developed between CAM and the hospital, and there was a culture clash between independent practitioners and team approaches to health and healing.

> The model was such a new model that patients weren't familiar with it. The model was, here is an internist, here is somebody who knows herbs and acupuncture and all these other things who will integrate everything. And the patients were used to going to their primary care physician for standard medicine. If they wanted acupuncture they went to an acupuncturist; if they wanted herbs they went to a traditional Chinese herbalist. They weren't used to one-stop shopping. And so it was a totally different model and they didn't really want to come for integration of all their medical needs. It was a difficult sell. [Administrator P6]

In retrospect, the business model was predicated on a concept—the blended model—that might not have been marketable to patients. The popularity of CAM is based partially on its difference from traditional medicine. Its ambience is antithetical to that of the hospital or medical center. But the center was never able to provide this ambience in the space it occupied. Furthermore, CAM patients typically do not think of going to a hospital for their care.

> I'm not sure we were meeting patients' needs. My supposition is that, for one reason or another, our product was not, on its own, attractive to patients.

> We built an Edsel. Good car, but it wasn't going to sell. [Administrator P12]

Financial Issues

One important advantage the administration had in setting up the center was that it could offer higher salaries.

> We were finding that there was a market interest in these kinds of physicians that would bump up the salaries closer to $200,000. We didn't have a structure for general internists for that, and there was no way to justify it. [Administrator P13]

Yet this advantage was partly nullified because, as a PC, the center was required to pay the hospital for its space and was required to use and pay for the hospital's billing services. In addition, although it was loosely housed under the umbrella of the hospital's medical system through the foundation, as a separate corporation, the center was not covered by the hospital's insurance. This meant that the center had to purchase separate plans to protect the providers and the PC owners.

Added to these unexpected start-up costs were the costs of higher-than-market salaries and inflexible labor contracts for the allied health providers, who were guaranteed full salaries regardless of whether they saw patients. Reimbursement for services rendered was low. Because of its low revenues, the center began paying allied health professionals an hourly rate. In contrast to the business model's projections, CAM providers were not being hired on as FTEs, and the center lacked the revenue to increase the number of full-time staff.

Differences in coding practice between clinicians and the billing office also created problems. While state regulations mandated the billing codes that could be reimbursed through insurance, the interpretation of and amendments made to the center's invoices by the hospital's billing services further limited reimbursement.

> The coding was one of the first issues. [In] the [billing] coding book it says exactly . . . what types of diagnoses . . . you have to have to be able to qualify . . . [so diagnoses need to be matched with the right codes, so the issue was] how do you maximize, legally, your profitability? The coders at [the hospital] didn't see

it in the same context as the [clinicians] who were providing the service. [Administrator P34]

The internal regulations and bureaucratic mechanisms, such as billing procedures and the requirement to accept both public and private insurance, may have introduced insurmountable barriers to the center's success.

The center's services, particularly the lengthy intake evaluation, restricted patient volume. While the original business plan included the equivalent of five full-time providers seeing patients six days a week, the center was top-heavy with physicians and CAM providers, while its patient base remained limited. The constricted revenue stream was compounded by the lack of spin-off income. The only means of creating this kind of "high-spark" income—herbs and pharmaceuticals—was moved to the hospital's pharmacy department. This choked off the only potential high-margin income for the IM center and undermined its profitability.

Adding to the problems, the original business plan, which was based on a cash-only outpatient center, was jettisoned. As an affiliate of the hospital, the PC was required to accept private health insurance.

In the outpatient model we originally created, we almost didn't care if insurance paid. The successful models we looked at in this area and around the country [were] cash-and-carry businesses. [Administrator P13]

In addition to accepting private health insurance, the center was required to accept Medicare and Medi-Cal, two low-reimbursement payer sources. Even though it was set up independently from the hospital, the center was serving hospital patients and, therefore, had to accept Medicare. This meant that the IM center billed Medicare and waited for payments. Also, it could only bill up to the amount Medicare would pay, and there was no guarantee Medicare would pay for the service at all. At successful IM centers, patients pay cash when services are rendered.

[The] process is very lengthy and has a lot of cost to it . . . . [Also,] they did no mathematical analysis on how many patients they would have to see at what I call the "Medicare rate" in order to pay this . . . . [L]et's say you're paying out at $70 an hour and your Medicare reimbursement is $50. Now you know how many patients you have to see at $50 in order to cover it. [Administrator P39]

Relying on the dominant payer pools of public and private insurance significantly decreased the viability of the center. Its profit margin was already small, and the lengthy and capitated reimbursement process for CAM/IM services further eroded profitability. The center eventually tried to shore up the PC's growing losses by requiring cash payments from patients. However, this did not help. Patients were reluctant to pay cash for their care, indicating that the hypothesized niche market was not there. The patients expected the payment schedule to be like that of the rest of the hospital. They were accustomed to presenting their insurance card, perhaps making a small co-payment, and getting care. The idea of paying out of pocket for services was an unpopular one among many patients.

So who does the hospital end up with? They end up with all these people, this 30, 50, whatever percent of people who want to try alternative medicine in a safe environment, and yet they don't want to pay for it. That's who you're getting here. You're not bringing additional people to your hospital. [IM Provider P11]

Because of the small number of inpatient services that the center provided, the insurance reimbursement was even more problematic. Many of these services were not reimbursed, and hospital patients are not likely to have their wallets with them when services are being rendered. Again, insurance may not cover these services; few CAM services—and even fewer inpatient CAM services—are reimbursed.

Finally, because the corporation was established as an "arm's length" PC, it lacked mechanisms to funnel revenue back into the hospital, which might have helped its sustainability.

The business plan also created major—and unexpected—costs, including the legal fees to create the center as a separate corporation and the cost of a broad array of medical and corporate insurance. For example, the hospital's malpractice insurance, which covers its faculty, did not extend to the IM center; and because the center was a "new concept," this insurance was high. In addition, because the center was hiring providers from outside the hospital, they were required to purchase "tail insurance" to cover patients they had previously treated. (Tail insurance covers the period after a physician leaves his or her previous practice; it covers those patients who may still pose a liability risk.) And once the PC owners discovered that they would be legally responsible for the corporation's finances, they also purchased expensive directors and officers (D&O) insurance to protect themselves from financial losses. If they had been hospital employees, their malpractice insurance would have been fully covered by the hospital.

The hospital's concerns about the center's medical liability in general were heightened by the marginal position of CAM in Euro-American biomedical institutions. These concerns extended to the issue of dispensing herbs through the center, which contributed to the decision to use the hospital pharmacy for these prescriptions, even though the sale of herbs could have benefited the center financially and might have made it a sustainable entity.

> You know who runs [the hospital]? Risk management. These guys have an umbrella organization that covers [the hospital], and all they have to say is "boo" and everybody stops what they're doing. [IM Provider P1]

Administrative Issues

Several administrative features facilitated the creation of the center. As we noted earlier, the mandate to be at the cutting edge led the planners to take a proactive stance toward exploring, developing, and promoting novel medical programs, such as integrating an IM center into a hospital setting.

The hospital's organizational culture places high value on intellectual openness, responsiveness to community needs, its community "roots," and entrepreneurship. CAM touched upon each of these values, as it required the hospital staff to be intellectually adventurous in being open to different medical models. This orientation also fostered attentiveness to the perceived community needs of patients "voting with their feet." [Administrator P27]

However, hospitals are highly bureaucratic institutions. Bureaucracy and turf issues—the hallmarks of most large corporations—also mark this institution, and the hospital moves slowly to implement new policies. Thus, while the hospital's ethos prizes innovation, hierarchies and turf issues impede risk taking, radical changes in culture, or challenges to existing political structures. As in most institutional environments, many of the ongoing struggles are not reactions to genuine threats but issues of ego and power.

There was high turnover in the clinic administrator position at the IM center. The first administrative director was an assistant to the hospital president and had been a member of the task force. Soon overwhelmed with the amount of work on this "special project," the director passed the job to another administrator, who was expected to weave together the three-part design of research, clinical, and education components. Unfortunately, this person had personal friction with several IM center staff members; the administrator departed and was not replaced. Instead, the operations manager, who was initially hired to help with a grant, stayed on to do day-to-day program administration.

The center came under a succession of hospital administrators, including the vice president of medical/surgery and the vice president of ambulatory care. But even with this train of managers, the amount of actual management provided was limited. Roles, obligations, and lines of authority were ill-defined, which made it difficult to run the center.

We didn't have a manager or an administrator who actually did any management or administration at any time that I was there. Some of that was because the job was never defined. The role was never defined. [Nor was it clear] who everyone was answerable to [in the] hierarchy. [IM Provider P29]

From an administrative point of view, the role of director of the center seemed unclear. The director had little, if any, authority and no power. For example, the director was not given reports about the center's financial status and was excluded from policymaking meetings, while the chair of the Department of Medicine and the senior vice president of medical affairs had the right to hire and fire staff and oversee fellows and residents.

Marketing/Public Relations

The center's viability was seriously undermined by the lack of a professional, coordinated, and sustained marketing and public relations campaign. The creators may have assumed that the hospital's prestigious reputation made such a campaign unnecessary; however, the lack of funding for marketing limited in-house acceptance of the center and impeded its ability to establish a referral and patient base.

In some ways, the reputation of the hospital worked against the center. As one respondent observed, part of the hospital's prestige rests on its cachet as a celebrity hospital, although a substantial number of patients are Medicare recipients.

I mean, 42 percent of the patients who come to [the hospital] are Medicare patients. We only get in the news . . . if X bumps her head. But the fact is, that's not all we do. [Administrator P7]

Even the few marketing efforts that were made faced internal impediments, including a reluctance to allow use of the hospital's brand. Some people feared that the well-respected and well-established brand would be jeopardized if it were linked to an IM clinic. At the same time, the hospital's high profile may have contributed to the perception that a marketing campaign for the center was unnecessary. The administration appears to have been confident that it could rely on name recognition. This overconfidence may also help explain why so little marketing research was conducted before the center was established to ensure that a niche market did, in fact, exist. Part of the problem on the marketing side was that integrative medicine was such a new model that patients were not familiar with it.

A related struggle was creating a marketable concept, label, and name for the center. How could a hospital that treats sick people be made to appear compatible with CAM's health and wellness orientation? The hospital had no previous experience with integration, so even deciding what to call the center was a challenge. Planners wrestled with basic questions: What do you call it? How does it interact with other disciplines? Is it medicine or not?

Part of the difficulty rested with its hospital affiliation, even though the center was located down the street. The public associates hospitals with sickness; people do not want to sit next to sick people to get their acupuncture or massage treatments.

> I mean, why would you come here for a massage? [Administrator P8]

In addition to these branding impediments, the hospital administration did not provide funding to market the center and placed restrictions on the kinds of marketing the center could do. Nonmainstream community venues were not considered appropriate, so the efforts of the center often conflicted with the hospital's marketing protocols. The center was not able to freely market its practice.

> I wanted to do some marketing in the health food stores, the herb places, places where the patients I want to see would be. I was told, "No, [the hospital] doesn't leave cards at grocery stores and drugstores." [IM Provider P43]

One perspective about the lack of marketing was that IM was not perceived as "A-list" material and was given low priority for any kind of coordinated, sustained public relations.

> I think the norm is not to market and push except for the trophy type of new programs. Dr. X is a solid brain tumor surgeon. You

can bet your bottom dollar that six-figure money was invested in marketing him. [Hospital Provider P45]

This comment illuminates the common protocol for marketing programs. It was not only the IM center that was let down by the system with regard to marketing; other centers did not get aggressive marketing either, compared with what the big moneymaking units received. The IM center was not totally neglected, but it was not on the A-list for marketing.

But the key factor was the nonexistent marketing budget. The hospital put its prestige on the line in approving and implementing an integrative medical clinic but did not showcase it. The lack of effective public relations or a genuine marketing campaign did not go unnoticed internally, where it was interpreted as a lack of support.

That's so typical of [the hospital]. They start something, they get it up and running, and they don't support it to let it really develop. [IM Provider P3]

The lack of public relations was confusing to some physicians, who assumed that they had not heard about the center because it was outside their department's purview. The marketing efforts (such as they were) were ineffective in targeting key players across the internal hierarchies and business divisions, and so did not overcome the balkanization that typically plagues large organizations.

I never got any type of literature. No one ever contacted me personally. I don't know exactly why. Maybe because it was through the Department of Medicine rather than the Department of Surgery. [Administrator P8]

The center's only brochure featured the IM physicians but excluded the CAM providers. This alienated the latter, despite the fact that the center had gone to significant lengths to secure an in-house credentialing program so these providers could be hired.

We didn't have a brochure for the first year. And when they came out with the brochure, who was in it? [Only the IM physicians.]

They didn't include any alternative practitioners in the brochure. It was a joke! [IM Provider P24]

Perhaps most important, the internal marketing campaign failed to win physician referrals. Some physicians were not only worried about financial competition; they were also concerned about protecting the hospital's brand as a prestigious "allopathic shop." A CAM/IM approach could be perceived not as a value-added option but as a threat to the traditional MD knowledge base and expertise.

Because the center was unable to effectively market itself internally across the hospital's business and hierarchical structures, it missed a significant opportunity: the 800-patient-a-day in-house population.

Those 800 patients—almost every one of them could use a consult. We have a lot of patients who use herbal medications. They just need a review leading up to surgery. Are they taking things that might complicate their surgical stay and increase their length of stay? The hospital missed a golden opportunity there. [Administrator P34]

Another missed opportunity was that the center failed to make use of available resources to solicit and secure donor funding. Unfortunately, when the second center director secured a viable donor, the funding ended up going to a competing in-house allopathic department. Possibly through an act of omission, the leadership of the hospital channeled a substantial donation from a satisfied IM center patient to go to a more powerful department.

In terms of image, the center lacked the spa-like ambience of local high-end CAM providers. It was small, cramped, and lacked visibility. Many wealthy people use CAM and IM, but the center was not attractive enough to those kinds of people that they would support it with donations.

The center's external marketing efforts lacked political savvy in terms of establishing both a referral and a patient base. First, it was unrealistically assumed that CAM providers in the community would be willing to refer a large volume of their patients to a hospital-based IM center. Second, the center spent some of its scant marketing resources giving lectures to communities that could not afford its services and persons who were unlikely to become patients.

> They were people who had way too much time on their hands and came for the [free] meal. [IM Provider P29]

Competition

The IM center faced unexpectedly strong external competition from private practices, local medical centers, and CAM businesses in its catchment area. And several factors influenced internal referrals, including the perceived "threat" posed by the center, a sense of competition among providers that typically occurs in the hospital setting, and some CAM services that already existed in the hospital.

Because the faculty relied on referrals from community doctors, they attempted to avoid aggravating them. This meant that the faculty tended not to practice specialties that might compete with community doctors. This was the nature of the environment the IM center was entering.

Perceived Threats

Stakeholder groups in a multistranded and hierarchical organization may perceive any new program or clinic as a threat. For example, even the Woman's Health Program—a paper-based screening program with no clinical component—was seen as a potential threat by some physicians. Despite having an endowed chair and a staff, it was not permitted to do any clinical work.

CAM is philosophically distinct from biomedicine; it has historically been perceived as "less than" and in conflict with western medical models. Thus, the center represented potential competition for the hospital's biomedical providers. At the same time, existing in-house allied health providers saw CAM not so much as "complementary" medicine but rather as less-well-trained competition. For example, the physical therapists looked down on chiropractors, acupuncturists, and massage therapists. Instead of seeing the CAM providers as "physician extenders," many people saw them as competition to medical practice.

> I remember when we had our first chiropractor . . . . I thought the orthopedic guys were going to go crazy. Low back pain. They thought, whoa, there goes that whole body of work. That's not what the chiropractors are here for, but they saw it as a threat. If it's a threat, you keep them out. [Administrator P66]

Allied health professionals viewed the IM center and CAM providers as potential competition. The threat was related to the perceived lack of training and licensure among CAM providers, especially when the services they provide, such as physical therapy, may look the same as what physical therapists do.

> If you have people at a lower level doing activities that look the same, then people think, well, it's no big deal, anybody can do it, whereas we're licensed to do it. [Administrator P78]

Generalists and primary care physicians seemed to feel more threatened by CAM than specialists did. This issue surfaced in referral practices among hospital physicians.

In addition to turf issues across medical hierarchies, the IM center model that was implemented, with its emphasis on an outpatient clinic rather than research, posed a structural problem. The faculty at the hospital was not expected to have outpatient clinics because they would compete with the private doctors, so the hospital did not have structures to support an outpatient clinic.

IM Center as Nonthreatening

Not all providers were wary of CAM; some saw the center as offering care that drew from a different market or provided services that were different enough to be nonthreatening.

> [The CAM provider] never takes over my patients and knows I want to take care of my own patients, because [the provider]

understands my side. [The provider] is not doing the same [thing] I'm doing anyway. [Hospital Provider P42]

Coexisting CAM

Numerous hospital departments provided some form of CAM services before and while the IM center was in operation. These units included cardiology departments, gastroenterology, a spine center, women's health/OB-GYN, psychiatry, and oncology, as well as orthopedics, a pain clinic, radiology, rehab, and urology. In cardiac surgery, for example, CAM included guided imagery, yoga, and acupuncture. These CAM services may have represented unwanted competition for the IM center.

Referrals

Attitudes toward the IM center as threatening, benign, or useful were manifested in descriptions of how and why hospital providers did or did not make referrals to the center. Only primary care physicians can make a referral to a *specific* physician. It may be that this prescribed behavior is even more pronounced with regard to making referrals outside the medical institution.

When a patient is referred, institutional norms obligate the provider who receives the referred patient to contact the referring physician to share information about findings and any treatment provided. This facilitates continuity of care. However, it is also a way to show deference to referring providers and assure them that their patients will not be "stolen." Providers who do not adhere to these prescribed behaviors will not receive patient referrals again. CAM providers were often perceived as violators of these referral norms.

> I take very good care of my patients and I need to know everything that's going on. The surgeons, when I send a patient to a surgery, know that if they don't call me and tell me what happened to that patient, what that patient's abdomen felt like in the OR, then they're never going to get a patient from me again. The acupuncturists and the chiropractors and the herbalists couldn't get this together, for them to understand that I am the primary

caretaker of this patient, and I know everything about everything, from psychologically to physically. [Hospital Provider P42]

I sent people to these alternative medicine providers, and they never told me what was going on. I think I'm pretty good at acupuncture, but I'm not great. So if I have somebody who's a really tough case, I'll refer them to an acupuncturist. But I've got to tell you, I'll never hear from them again. [Hospital Provider P42]

CAM providers in the center were aware of this issue. They knew that some physicians thought they stole patients, but most took care to ensure that any test results were sent to the referring physician and all patients were returned to their primary care doctors.

This issue of patient "ownership" has at least two additional dimensions. First, there are turf issues. Do the CAM services encroach on the referring provider's turf, whether in terms of treatment and services provided or hospital privileges? Second, has the CAM provider received in-house credentialing that delegitimizes or competes with the referring provider's training or licensure? The hospital's physical therapists, for example, believed that their training and expertise could be jeopardized if the IM center hired movement therapists.

Some of the hospital's physicians have reputations as adamant "patient owners." Moreover, managed care, with its structure of primary care physicians as gatekeepers, in essence mandates and validates a culture of patient ownership. The situation got complicated when patients requested that the IM provider become their primary care provider.

If it's a physician that they know wants total control and the patient is asking, even at that extreme point we would still say, "Go back to your primary." [Administrator P78]

From the beginning, the IM center was presented as a consultative practice, partially to circumvent patient ownership issues. The developers characterized the practice as not interested in long-term primary care medicine and said all referrals would be returned. They assumed, however, that the center would also draw referrals from community CAM providers in the hospital's catchment area. Neither of these aspects of the plan was realized.

It was assumed that the director's training as an internist would help address concerns about referrals. That is, the director would be culturally astute and would not provide or suggest treatment that would be considered too extreme or threatening to the biomedical model in a prestigious hospital, and referral norms would be observed.

> I send someone to a chiropractor, I never see them again. They're getting their neck and back manipulated, the chiropractor's putting them on yeast therapy . . . let me tell you as a physician, through some of the experiences I've had with CAM practitioners, they're doing things way beyond CAM. [Expert P37]

There is a perception among physicians that if they send patients to a CAM provider, they're going to do all kinds of "wacky stuff" and they'll never see the patient again. But in this case, they knew that the director had the same medical background as they did. The CAM provider would help the patient, sort out the alternative modalities the patient was using or could use, and then send the patient back.

> That was the promise that was made. The marketing message to the practitioners was, "You send them to me, you're not going to lose them. I'm with you on the medical stuff, but I'm going to start doing all this other stuff to help your patients feel better." [Expert P37]

However, having internists on staff proved to be both a barrier to the center's success and one of its strongest facilitators. IM center internists were viewed as bicultural and, therefore, able to translate CAM to biomedical providers. In particular, the center director and the fellows (who had received their training at this hospital) were perceived as speaking the same language as the hospital's biomedical providers. But having bicultural internists—and therefore generalists rather than medical specialists—created a barrier to the center's success, because generalists tend to "own" their patients.

I don't think we got a lot of referrals from physicians. I think that may be in part because, despite our efforts to calm the concerns . . . , people may have worried that we would be stealing their patients. If an internist refers to an acupuncturist, the acupuncturist isn't going to be providing internal medicine services. However, if you refer to our program, we've got an internist who's also in the program. So I think there were some questions as to what they were referring to, and if they were asked in the first place, why wouldn't they refer to an acupuncturist they trusted? [Administrator P12]

Most patients believe they have a right to choose their primary care physician. Thus, some hospital physicians thought the presence of internists at the center increased the likelihood that patients might go there and stay there. The result was that patients who liked the IM approach and wanted something that was not so mainstream found that they were unable to convert to the center for primary care. In trying to allay the fears of the referring physicians, IM center doctors antagonized the patients who valued the service most.

Referral Sources
How were patients referred to the IM center? The director brought a few patients and the hospital's call center provided some referrals; but the two main sources were word of mouth among the patients and hospital physician referrals. The oncology, cardiac, and gastroenterology departments made multiple referrals, but these were often patient-driven—providers were simply the necessary conduits to patients' obtaining an IM center referral.

If you want to take a proportion of how many I send by self-referral versus [by my] suggesting, I think it's probably 90 percent self-referral, meaning the patient has heard of [them] or I'm sending because my methods are failing, versus me using it as first line. [Hospital Provider P46]

However, some providers in these departments did make multiple referrals to the center. One of the respondents describes the informal process of building a referral network with the center director.

> Somewhere along the line I knew that [the center] existed, and I think I called [one of the providers] about a patient. Then I know there were one or two or three patient interactions, and the office was over in a building where I also go from time to time because of another program [there], and I ducked down and introduced myself. That gave the collegial connection which allowed them to say, "Oh, you're X. I'm Y. Hi." Turned out to be an interesting person, and we began to have a relationship. [Hospital Provider P49]

Other physicians began making referrals to the center through a more formal process. Because previous interest in CAM overlapped with one physician's expertise, he collaborated on a grant with the IM center director. This led to referrals from this physician to the IM center. For other providers, the fact that the center was hospital-based was the key facilitating factor. In other words, these providers were more comfortable making an in-house CAM referral.

One referral source that did not develop at all was that of the surrounding CAM providers, who were uninformed about the center, had referral networks of their own, or saw the center as competition.

Referral Characteristics

Some hospital physicians referred directly to the IM providers, while others emphasized keeping business in-house.

> The allegiance I had to [a local school of Oriental medicine], which is where I was sending my patients, was zero. I'm a [hospital] guy, and I said, "I'll send you whatever I can." [Hospital Provider P45]

Physicians were most likely to refer patients suffering from chronic conditions. Some referred by CAM modality or to a specific CAM provider. Knowing and trusting the IM provider was important but, again, many referrals were patient-driven. Others referred specific types of patients: the "worried well" and the "difficult" patient, the ones with a litany of complaints.

The impact of this "dumping" cannot be underestimated. Patients who did not respond to conventional therapies were time drains for hospital physicians, who were glad to have a place to send them. Thus, the IM center's patient base from hospital referrals was partly a population of nonresponsive patients. Further, it was not uncommon for a referred patient to bring bags full of herbal supplements to the first appointment, requiring several (unbillable) hours to sort through.

Physicians also may have made patient-driven referrals for those seeking a "natural" approach. But one of the key factors in building a referral base may have been establishing reciprocal referrals; that is, referring IM center patients to hospital providers. The complex way in which referrals occurred, even with a single physician, is captured in the quote below:

> I had a few patients in common with [the IM center] who, when they felt that they needed more of our regular medication, then they would come to me. And so they would be on a host of their medications and a few of ours. I don't have enough evidence yet to say that because they were on those, I had to give less doses. But at least I know it didn't hurt them. I get lots of patients, especially in this area where everybody wants to be "natural," who actually want to use the techniques. I tend to send them to [the IM center] because I know that the two physicians that I work with have trained with me. We're pretty much contemporaries. And another group of patients [that] I tend to send [are], for example, pain patients. Or they're older, fragile people who have severe osteoarthritis. I tend to send to them because they've tried everything or they've got kidney dysfunction and they can't use our regular medication . . . so that's another reason why I use [the IM center at the hospital, because at least I know who these people are. I know it's not "voodoo medicine." I know I can call them any time and vice versa. [Hospital Provider P46]

Patient Expectations

The most common expectation patients expressed was simply "to feel better" or to get better. Others explicitly sought an integrative approach or a primary care provider with an integrative medical perspective. A few patients said they had no expectations.

Center Met Their Expectations

When asked if their experience at the center met their expectations, more than half responded that it had; they appreciated the amount of time that they were given, the care they received, feeling better, and, for some, being able to avoid taking pharmaceutical drugs.

> It exceeded my expectations just by how much time she took with me and the care. How she went over everything and how much effort she put into it. By getting me on track and making me stronger. I feel that helped a lot. [IM Patient P38]

The vast majority of patients reported positive experiences with their provider. Again, their comments focused on the amount of time and the quality of care they received. These two factors were followed by comments about providers' knowledge of CAM, and the fact that the IM approach fostered a sense of personal responsibility for their own health and hope.

> I like the fact that I never felt rushed by the doctor. And it was small enough that everybody seemed to know you and everybody seemed very concerned about me. I didn't feel as though I was being talked down to or patronized in any way, and I felt that I was part of my own healing. Part of the program was that I was responsible for healing myself. [IM Patient P8]

Most patients said their treatment had been helpful, either in promoting their health from a mechanistic perspective or on a mind-body level. In fact, some patients raved about the difference that the care they received at the center had made in their lives or their illness experience.

Their support made everything bearable. I can say that. I don't know how I would have managed. Because it was connected with the hospital in that way, it made it painless to find out about how to . . . manage everything. It was all a package. I consider the holistic, the eastern methods, but I do the western as well. The balance is what I think helped me. I felt like I was in control of my health. [IM Patient P22]

Center Did Not Meet Their Expectations

Almost a third of the patients, however, said that the IM center did not meet their expectations. A few patients said they expected the ability of the center to meet their expectations to improve as it became more established, but it decreased over time as the center was downsized.

Initially, I had the sense that it was a good beginning effort but not meeting my full expectations. But I continued to have an expectation that that would continue to improve, that [the center] was really just getting off the ground. But as time went on, my expectations have been decreased because of the changes in the organization of the clinic, and what appears to be the support that the medical center gives to it, so that in the course of the last several years it has barely met my expectations. But again, I want to make clear that I lay the responsibility for that with the hospital, not with the staff of the clinic itself. [IM Patient P19]

The patients who were not satisfied with the treatments they received generally were disappointed because they felt that one or more of their treatments lacked efficacy, that the center's range of treatment alternatives was limited, or that the treatments were not aggressive enough (e.g., compared with previous Korean acupuncture treatments).

While the majority of the patients were satisfied with the support staff, some were less than generous in their evaluations, and one respondent called the staff "very unprofessional."

Would They Refer Others?

The most telling evaluation of any medical model is whether patients deem their care or provider worthy of referring to others. One of the most positive evaluations of the IM center is that patients overwhelmingly reported that they had referred or would refer someone. The two most common reasons for their enthusiastic endorsement were that the center's approach went beyond the limitations of western medicine and to make a referral to their specific provider.

> I would have no problem referring anybody. I've spoken very fondly [to others] about that center because I thought they did a lot for me. I think that there are times when ordinary medicine doesn't quite do it. I think it's wonderful to have a place like the center for alternative methods of treatment. [IM Patient P18]

Given the significant prestige of the hospital, it was striking that only one patient mentioned the hospital's reputation as a reason for making a referral. Moreover, only a few patients said they would make a referral because of the quality or perceived efficacy of the care they received.

It was not uncommon for respondents to mention a caveat when we discussed referral. Over a fourth of the patients expressed reservations about recommending the center because of the lack of availability of the providers and the difficulty of getting an appointment. Only a few patients said they would not refer anyone to the center. Their dissatisfaction had to do with a perceived deficient range of services or quality of the providers.

Research and Training Issues

The center's training and research components were eclipsed by its emphasis on clinical care. While the training efforts began even before the center opened, they were overshadowed by an emphasis on patient care and increasing patient volume. Research efforts grew over time. Although the environment was fairly receptive and the timing for CAM/IM research and education was good, these components were hindered primarily by the lack of staff with strong academic research experience and enough seniority to oversee fellowship training. Other barriers, such as burdensome internal and external regulations, might have been overcome if the center had had the time, personnel, and funding necessary to grow a CAM/IM research and training agenda, but it had none of those.

Unlike many academic medical centers, this hospital's primary focus is clinical care rather than teaching or research. This made the "fit" of an IM model within this private hospital setting more problematic.

> There is research happening here. It's encouraged and supported to a good extent, especially considering [that] this is a nonuniversity private hospital. I don't know that there's another one that even comes close to this one in terms of the amount of research that goes on broadly. But it arises from the individuals here who want to do the research. The majority of [the hospital] is still very good, private practicing doctors who are delivering good, standard care to their patients in an environment that tries to make every effort to make the delivery of care paramount. [Hospital Provider P87]

Other hospital programs had successful research programs that the center hoped to piggyback on or emulate.

The research component faced significant barriers in testing herbs and supplements. The time needed for a small start-up enterprise—to write successful grants and secure funding—was not included in the business model. Moreover, even with funding, this kind of outside-the-box research faces the external barriers of a protracted FDA approval process. As one of the respondents noted, these kinds of obstacles require staff who are willing to swim upstream against the odds.

Physicians' hubris regarding their own research abilities also becomes problematic in academic medicine environments. So while the problems the center faced were not unusual, they were amplified by the research agenda and the type of physicians and providers involved.

> That is a very astute observation of almost all hospitals. I see people being hired into chief of medical affairs positions, the heads of

quality improvement who have never published a paper in their life and are expected to evaluate huge programs within hospitals. They have no idea what they're going to do. It's a generic phenomenon outside of academic institutions. In fact, it's very consistent with how the hospital operates. [Expert P37]

In addition to these impediments to success, the research and teaching components of the IM center model, similar to those of the clinical component, suffered from a lack of space. This problem was endemic to the hospital.

Besides the lack of physical space, the IM director was not given "space" within the hospital as an appointed faculty member. The hospital's faculty undergoes an internal review process for appointment. A successful candidate who would like to teach is offered an additional appointment as an assistant professor at a local university that houses a medical school. A potential barrier to the center's success was that its director was not given an academic appointment. While the director retained a faculty position at another local university, the lack of an in-house identity as a hospital faculty member diminished any gravitas the director brought to the role as center director.

Research Program

The original research plan was to set up the center to collect outcomes data on its patients. This plan was not implemented because of budget constraints.

The staff's research and teaching experience was uneven, at best. The fellows were, understandably, still acquiring research and teaching skills. The first fellow had previous training in health services research, but the other fellows did not possess the skills necessary to conduct research. But the most significant staff problem as far as securing grant funding was the director's lack of research experience.

The center encountered other obstacles to securing research funding, including navigating the hospital's bureaucratic structure in a timely fashion.

It took the Grants and Contracts Department seven months to dicker around with the lawyers. The funding was gone by the time they agreed to sign the contract. That was a $100,000 grant that didn't materialize because they couldn't execute it. [IM Provider P4]

The director joined a research team at another institution for a large NCCAM proposal that had been awarded funding and also began to develop research projects with other colleagues outside the center.

IM and CAM research faces the obstacles of Internal Review Boards (IRBs) and external FDA regulations. In addition, Health Insurance Portability and Accountability Act (HIPAA) regulations, which slow down most patient-based medical research, went into effect just as the center was established. This created yet another impediment to the center's ability to quickly design and establish research projects, better secure its research projects' financial status, or establish a successful research foundation.

> What we really wanted was herb . . . research. Our irritable bowel disease people collected 40 of these patients, worked it out so they'd study these herbs, and then put in through our IRB. Our IRB said, "Well, it's true that these things are over the counter and anybody can walk in and get them, but now you're using it to treat a disease and therefore it's classified as a drug and you have to get an IND [investigational new drug] application from the FDA." So we put in for an IND with the FDA, and the FDA said, "Well, if you're going to get an IND, you have to do all this toxicology study and all this other stuff," and nobody wanted to pay for that, so it became a catch-22. [Administrator P6]

Another barrier to integrating research and training in a hospital-based IM environment (which other IM centers have had to overcome) is the association of CAM with wellness and as a means of reducing, not inducing, stress. Patients typically do not associate CAM treatments with becoming a research participant, so they were surprised by these requests. In this center, the questionnaire that was designed to collect patient data on intake was 12 pages long.

You send them a 12-page document to fill out, and they're like, "Eeek, I don't want to go. Why should I go there?" And sometimes people would make appointments, they'd send them the materials and they'd call up and cancel. I don't want to go to the doctors and have a fellow standing in the room while I'm being examined, being taught what's going on with my treatment . . . . For your acupuncture, do you want someone standing over you while they're putting the needles in you and saying, "I'm using this spot because this does what?" That's not relaxing to me as the patient who's lying on the table. [Administrator P8]

Resistance to CAM

The center's creators believed that they would encounter opposition to the establishment of a hospital program incorporating CAM, particularly from the medical staff. Given the historical animosity between biomedicine and CAM, this was a reasonable assumption. An important and interesting result of this case study is that the expectation of opposition was largely not met. The responses varied from supportive to open opposition, but there was not enough of the latter to create a movement to halt operations.

The hospital's ethos, which supports institutional innovation and cultural openness, helped mitigate resistance to the IM center. In fact, CAM was already being used by small pockets of the medical staff.

I thought the medical staff here, notwithstanding their strong skepticism, as a whole showed a remarkable amount of neutrality at least and even support for the chairman and his effort to do this. And then within the medical staff, there were pockets of people who were already actively engaged [in CAM]. [Administrator P27]

Lack of financial support beyond the initial seed money turned out to be a more significant problem than opposition from biomedicine. The hospital is as much a bottom-line business as it is an innovative institution, particularly in lean economic times. Closing the IM center (described in the following section) was not based on resistance; rather, it was a pragmatic business decision. As one administrator pointed out, economics—not culture—sealed the center's fate. However, the lack of financial support might be interpreted as reflecting high levels of skepticism about CAM among the hospital's physicians and executive administrators.

> Maybe [they were] a little skeptical, more so on [Dr. X]'s part I think than [the chairman of the Department of Medicine]'s, but a little skeptical about the real value of it, but willing to try it. And open to it. But when the going got tough, [it was] "Let's get rid of it." [Administrator P52]

It is also critical to note that little active resistance should not be interpreted as *no* resistance. Resistance to CAM ranged from hostility to skepticism. The difficulty of translating and bridging the disparate cultures of biomedicine and CAM contributed to this resistance. Yet, many physicians are aware of the relatively high proportion of their patients who use CAM, and some providers saw it as a means of potentially broadening their own practice or clinic.

> There's a clear minority who strongly are in favor of using non-traditional therapies [who] bring it up to patients all the time. Then there's a group, maybe a strong minority, that is dissenting and really will be verbally caustic about any information that the patient may bring that they're trying [CAM]. That . . . makes the patients unwilling to discuss it with their physician. Then, a lot of people, the majority at least, half the oncologists and physicians, are in the middle. [Hospital Provider P72]

Those who were opposed to CAM and to attempts at integration were quite vociferous about it but did not seem to organize any opposition to the center's creation.

> Then there was this controversial minority that just weren't wowed with the thing. So it was pretty amazing. There was a lot of positive "Wow," but there was a really vocal minority who were negative. As it turns out, people were just having conniptions over

the whole concept. Some of them likened it to voodoo medicine, and some of them were concerned that [CAM] was untested and unproven. And that it was just counter [biomedicine] bothered people as much as anything. But that was a minority, and in general there was a surprising amount of interest in the whole area. The positive side is, by this time, I had realized that there were a lot of patients taking the stuff. So you might as well hop on board. [Administrator P94]

While the quotes above suggest that those who were resistant were vocal, data suggest that those either open to CAM or hostile to it were in the minority; the majority of physicians and providers were skeptical. They were uncertain about CAM and its place in this hospital or in their own practice.

Those who were opposed assumed that the majority felt the same way. The most common derisive descriptors were from those hostile to a nonbiomedical approach. They characterized CAM as a "joke" or likened it to something foreign, like "voodoo," "mumbo-jumbo" without scientific efficacy, a kind of "hocus-pocus." But even some of this group saw it as harmless.

However, part of the opposition was that this program was, in effect, taking away funding from some of the programs they had in mind.

Clinicians' overt hostility surprised some of their colleagues, but it may have been the covert hostility, such as that described below, that contributed to the hospital's lack of financial support for the center and to its ultimate demise by limiting its ability to develop a strong referral base.

Unfortunately, I've been vindicated, and I've taken a back seat. I haven't actively tried to close the program. I haven't actively had any [feed]back from the program, and I've not actively taken any public stand. I've been very quiet. I've purposely kept very quiet and just watched it evolve and basically self-destruct. [Administrator P44]

Other respondents believed that certain board members had foisted the center on a nonreceptive and skeptical hospital staff who were wary of CAM's efficacy and questioned its role in the hospital. There was also a suspicion that other members of the board did not favor the program and did not think it matched the prestige of the hospital but bowed to the pressure from the other board members.

Factors Influencing Physician Resistance

Age

Respondents noted two physician characteristics associated with resistance to CAM—age and medical specialty—although both categories are fuzzy. Some respondents believed that older physicians were more likely to be resistant or hostile to CAM, while others believed that the more experienced providers were more likely to be receptive to CAM. Overall, the responses suggest that the former assumption may be more accurate.

> At one of the very first conferences [the director] gave, one of the people who's been on the medical staff for years and has been a leader, is really involved and knows everybody, was standing outside the room saying, "This is all bullshit!" And the reaction that X got absolutely surprised me because the room was just split. Either this was nonsense or this was something interesting they wanted to learn about. [Hospital Provider P73]

> The real vocal ones tended to be the older guys. I think probably because they're not afraid to be really vocal about it and were a little more set in their ways. [Administrator P94]

Specialty

Surgeons and anesthesiologists were the most skeptical about integrating CAM because of potential negative interactions, especially during medical interventions. Internists, gynecologists, and pain clinic participants were more open to CAM modalities. While some oncologists were open to CAM, others thought it had a limited role in cancer care because of concerns about patient vulnerability. Pharmacists appear to be split in their attitudes.

> As a surgeon, I think the net issue is that it's harmful at its best. I'm talking against it specifically as a surgeon because we do invasive procedures and the bleeding issues are real major issues for us. Any potential advantage that patients are getting is far outweighed by the potential disadvantages. [Hospital Provider P93]

> For the most part, alternative therapy has been the bane of the existence in people who take care of cancer patients, because the general feeling is that they prey on the false hopes of patients and suck their wallet out because of it, and that has always been a predominant activity of these types of people. However, there is a middle ground with some people who have had cancer and want to be or are cancer-free who are looking for every type of medical and nonmedical management that they can find to make themselves healthy. And in that regard, there is a very solid place for alternative medicines and alternative therapies. [Hospital Provider P77]

Safety and Liability

Concerns about patient safety also raise issues of medical liability, which contributes to physician wariness about CAM. Their skepticism may be further amplified by concerns about their own image and the possibility of being labeled too "CAM-like" in a medical culture with fairly rigid ideologies about models of illness and healing, and appropriate practices. Some providers discouraged their patients because of the risks involved, particularly from herbal substances that can affect organs such as the liver. Pharmacists worried about these interactive effects and the fact the CAM substances are largely unregulated.

Efficacy

Lack of established "scientific" efficacy of CAM was a factor in many physicians' resistance to the IM center, although safety rather than efficacy was the dominant concern of the skeptics. Yet, as one respondent pointed out, biomedicine does not have a stronger track record than CAM of protecting its patients from harm.

> I actually think it's a perception on the part of the MDs, that chiropractors are less than qualified to be adjusting someone's neck. They don't understand chiropractic. They don't like it. They have fears about it because they don't really understand it. You've heard the horror stories. I have to say that I've heard more horror stories about MDs than I have about alternative medicine practitioners. One in four patients died because of drug interaction administered by MDs. So let's talk about the reality of who's really harming whom. But it is a perception. [Administrator P65]

Culture

Related to perceptions of CAM as dangerous are cultural differences, including the difference between biomedical and CAM training. As the following quotes illustrate, there is a huge divide at this level. It was partially overcome in the center because the leaders were western-trained physicians who had turned to CAM and could therefore speak both languages.

> I do know of MDs who dispense herbs, but my impression is [that] most of the community thinks those are flaky people. They don't embrace them as real doctors. [Hospital Provider P45]

There is a strong belief that there is a lot of quackery in the area of CAM. The fact that most providers are not MDs or are MDs from other countries is a barrier.

> If there's no science—even though there may be a huge social experience or epidemiologic experience, but there's really no written science to back it up—people are very skeptical. So our training kind of gets in the way of this as well. [Hospital Provider P73]

The culture of biomedicine, with the lengthy and rigorous training its members undergo, may make them wary of "outsiders." Similarly, its language creates a barrier between the two cultures. This was a challenge for the CAM providers when they presented in hospital grand rounds. They wanted the western-trained doctors to become more familiar with the philosophy, language, and diagnoses of the alternative paradigms.

> And I really wanted to be a part of that process, where western and eastern doctors feel much more comfortable with each other. That never happened. [IM Provider P24]

This lack of a shared paradigm around diagnoses was seen as causing difficulties with patients.

> They really hate [it] when they diagnose a problem, and [the patient then goes] to a complementary practitioner, and they say, "Oh, no, that's not what you have. You have this." Let's say they get sent in for an L4 right radiculopathy to the acupuncturist. And they've written on there, "L4 radiculopathy." And the acupuncturist says, "Well, you have a yin-deficient kidney." That may be true from a Chinese medicine perspective, but the patient will go back to the MD and say, "You told me I had an L4 radic. I have a kidney problem." And the MD hears about kidney, they think they have kidney stones. There's great miscommunication. The patient's upset, so the doctor gets upset, and that's the last referral that acupuncturist is going to get. There's a political piece, there's a protocol and communication piece that has to get done that isn't being done. [Hospital Provider P57]

Again, violations of social norms were likely to increase resistance to CAM, as when an IM provider failed to make follow-up calls to the referring physician. These kinds of social and cultural missteps decrease physicians' trust in CAM and its providers.

Culture was also significant for the CAM providers who were hired to work in the center. The hospital was a foreign environment to many of them. They often did not know the language, rituals, or culture of the hospital, or the proper procedures and protocols. The process is one of acculturation. But there is difficulty in accepting another culture's views of what constitutes curative or acceptable medicinal media. To many physicians, the herbs used in traditional Chinese medicine were seen as disgusting, if harmless.

Another significant culture clash was between CAM and the increasingly dense bureaucracy of biomedical institutions, which are resistant to change. In an elite medical institution, even one that prides itself on innovation, change is incremental and slow. Most CAM providers have worked, or do work, in small clinics rather than large bureaucratic institutions.

In addition to the difficulties of working within a bureaucratic structure, integrating CAM in this risk-adverse institutional environment raised issues about medical and financial liability. This institution (like most hospitals) is very conservative, and liability is a huge issue. If an acupuncturist punctures a patient's lung in a hospital, the hospital is going to get sued along with the acupuncturist.

The perception that the hospital had initiated an alliance for profit with a marginal medical practice like CAM also fueled resistance and skepticism about the IM center.

> I think the perception of a lot of physicians when this program was started was it was just the administration's attempt to make a quick buck on the latest trend. In some ways, it diminished the traditional medicine history of the hospital. I think a large number of people feel or felt that way. [Hospital Provider P82]

Expectations of Resistance

Skepticism, rather than active resistance, characterized the majority response to the IM center. The task force leaders had anticipated resistance among medical staff to integrating CAM within the hospital. Their "Trojan horse" approach was to identify and recruit opponents to the task force, thereby "converting" key personnel who might stand in the way of establishing the IM center.

However, the task force did not encounter problems securing support for the center, especially during the internal review processes. Task force members were surprised at how easily the project went through the process. As noted earlier, the MEC did not raise serious objections. The most common attitude was "wait and see."

However, the developers continued to expect a backlash, and protecting the center from this backlash was a key reason given for setting it up as a PC. The PC model superseded the research-focused model that the MEC and the board had approved, which had significant consequences in terms of their continued support for the center.

> They made a huge mistake from the beginning. They set it up as a separate company, because they were afraid of a backlash and this was a way for certain individuals to protect themselves from the backlash. But there was no backlash, because everyone just assumed it was a department in the hospital, so it wasn't affecting anyone. There was no negative impact. [Administrator P32]

The continued expectation of resistance from staff physicians may also have had a negative impact on the center's in-house marketing strategies. They marketed to interns, perhaps thinking that orthopedic surgeons and neurosurgeons would be totally opposed to chiropractors or herbalists treating someone with an abnormal MRI.

Overcoming Resistance: Changing Attitudes

Many respondents said their initial skepticism about CAM and the IM center changed over time. Factors that increased receptivity to CAM included personal experience, being a younger physician, and the scientific dissemination of information about CAM, either through grand rounds or through articles in respected medical journals; for example, the 1993 article by Eisenberg and colleagues in the *New England Journal of Medicine.*

> Older men [are most resistant to CAM]. But then, most of the doctors at [the hospital] are older men. Certainly the female physicians were, in general, more welcoming . . . . Most of the literature on physician attitudes [at] that time [said] the younger someone was, the more receptive they were. Females were more receptive, minorities were more receptive. People with personal experience were more accepting. [IM Provider P5]

Conforming to the rituals of biomedicine—such as publishing in medical journals—and, in particular, being attentive to the rituals of academic medicine helped build the credibility of the IM center. For example, the most common mode of introducing cutting-edge techniques and new findings, other than publishing, is through grand round presentations. The director's use of grand rounds was an effective way of introducing in-house staff to the IM center and to alternative approaches to health and healing.

> I think they're much more receptive now [and what helped was] them presenting to us and showing us some evidence. [The IM center director] became quite known amongst all of us very soon because of medical grand rounds and cardiology grand rounds. All of us were just like, "Wow." We had no idea that this department existed, and we had no idea what medications there were and what they did. [Hospital Provider P46]

> Basically, it was something that I developed a liking for once it got started. I had come from the old school where a lot of this stuff was voodoo, but this is something that when it was presented to me, it became really fascinating. [Provider P68]

In addition, experience with CAM—personally or through friends, family, or anecdote—also made people less wary of nonbiomedical approaches. Quite often this occurred when family members were treated successfully by CAM providers.

> I've seen [it] with my mother, who was cured of psoriasis. [H]er dermatologist said, "It's a chronic condition, you have to live with it for the rest of your life, there's no cure as yet, just don't get stressed out." And her hands would bleed, she couldn't drive, sometimes she couldn't cook because she never knew when it would flare up. She went to this homeopath and in less than two years she's cured . . . it's been seven years and [it's] never come back. [Administrator P20]

Openness to CAM

The key factors respondents associated with openness to CAM were experience with and knowledge about CAM, a physician's area of expertise, perceived patient demand, and a patient-centered perspective. Some respondents believed that (in contrast to certain earlier statements) older, more knowledgeable physicians were less resistant, along with those educated about CAM and those who had used CAM themselves. One respondent said it was a matter of degree of exposure and, in this case, location in a state where CAM is prevalent.

> It's lack of education. The MD who has more knowledge in it is more apt to say, "Okay, I think we can try this," or "I've had a patient who's benefited from this." [Provider P69]

As we know from the patient data below, physicians who treat chronic conditions such as fibromyalgia, irritable bowel syndrome, and colitis are more likely to be open to CAM, as are some pharmacists.

> Inflammatory bowel, Crohn's disease, ulcerative colitis—there's no real medical cure for these diseases. Surgically, you can, in a sense, cure ulcerative colitis by removing the colon, but even then some patients get prediagnosed with Crohn's disease. A lot of the medications don't work very well. Personally, I've always been open to alternative medical interventions. So we had some patients who wanted to try alternative therapy, because they want to try everything. There's one particular combination of herbal interventions that really seems to work in patients with ulcerative colitis. [Administrator P81]

Some practitioners were receptive to CAM because of its potential to provide additional streams of revenue.

Finally, physicians who perceived CAM providers as specialists rather than as part of an alternative medical system were more likely to accept CAM, particularly if the CAM providers were willing to follow normative referral patterns. The decision to refer a patient to a CAM specialist depends, as well, on the patient's receptivity. The downside of a physician being open to CAM (a minor theme in the findings above) is the risk to a physician's reputation in referring a nonreceptive patient; that is, if the patient thinks homeopathy is hocus-pocus, the physician might lose credibility by recommending this treatment.

Consumer demand for health care options, such as CAM, was another factor respondents associated with physician openness to CAM. Physicians were increasingly being asked about CAM, as often as several times a day. Also, research being published about the use of CAM was having an impact.

> David Eisenberg's lecture had a big [impact on my becoming more open to CAM] in terms of the number of people who were using it and the potential value of it. I thought to myself, "If this many people are using it, and yet they're not telling their physician, wouldn't there be value in a physician who could actually understand this stuff and be able to relate to their patients in these fields?" And then I started doing some critical appraisal of the literature and found that there is some merit to this. There was some chiropractic work by some [local] folks. [IM Provider P11]

It appears that the more patient-centered a biomedical provider is, the more likely he or she will be open to CAM. As the following quote shows, this could occur in the least expected places in medicine.

> Dr. [X] . . . pioneered this program in cardiothoracic surgery, because he knew himself . . . how relaxing a massage is and how that translates to less pain [and] . . . better healing. [Or] how acupuncture can help. In cardiac surgery, you would think that pain might be the number one complaint, but it wasn't. There were a handful of complaints that always came up: insomnia, lack of appetite, fatigue. Those were the first three big things. Pain was in there, sometimes first but not always. And how acupuncture could help patients sleep better. He knew the value of all that. So he was really the person who championed it the most. [Hospital Provider P48]

A similar situation was reported for cancer patients. Usually, it was the patient who initiated the use of CAM, and in most cases it was an additional treatment. For some patients, CAM provided emotional support; for others, it was related to treatment side effects. Certain kinds of patients want to be more actively involved in their own care, and choosing CAM empowers them. The IM center had institutional and academic credibility, as opposed to an individual alternative medicine practitioner. And it was convenient for the patients' physicians to have an IM center as part of the hospital.

Patient Reactions to Physician Resistance: Stigma and Nondisclosure

Our data support previous findings that patients' fear of being judged negatively by their biomedical providers increases the likelihood that they will withhold information about their CAM use. This can be overcome by the physician.

> When you tell them that you're into it, then all the stuff comes out. They say, "I've tried this, I've tried that." You get the whole story. I think they're embarrassed, and they think that I'm resistant. That I'm traditional medicine and I will think less of them. That I'll think I will not be able to take care of them because they're not going to do what I tell them to do, because what I'm going to tell them to do is going to be western medicine. I think that there is an embarrassment that what they're doing is voodoo. But you know, the voodoo sometimes works. [Hospital Provider P86]

In many cases, physicians believe their patients are not using CAM when, in fact, they have just not asked them about it.

Patients' Experience

Ultimately, the experience of the patients determined whether they returned to the center and told others about it; thus, we tried to ascertain the nature of that experience.

Physical Access

One of the things we wished to determine was the distance the patients traveled to receive care. Most patients reported traveling less than 30 minutes, or under 20 miles, to visit the IM center. Only one reported traveling at least an hour.

We were also interested in how easy it was for them to use the center. Parking at the first site was easy, especially as the IM center had validated parking at the beginning. But while many patients reported that parking was not a problem, some complained about the difficulty of finding a place to park in the "mess" of hospital parking and of the high cost of parking.

Some of the patients reported having difficulty finding the center once they arrived at the hospital. Most of these complaints related to the center's second and third sites and reflect the typical frustration of trying to find a physician or clinic for the first time at a large hospital. However, these difficulties were exacerbated by a lack of signage after the center moved into the hospital.

Patient Appointments

Most patients reported that it was easy to make an appointment at the IM center, although some complained about having to leave a message—sometimes multiple messages—instead of being connected to a receptionist. The second most common complaint was a particular doctor's limited availability. While most patients were able to make an appointment within one to three weeks, some reported having to wait a month or more. Making appointments become more problematic as the center was increasingly downsized.

Once patients arrived for their appointment, the waiting time was generally 20 minutes or less. Patients reported spending varying lengths of time with their provider, depending on the type of visit (e.g., initial intake, acupuncture, follow-up consultation). Most reported that contact with the provider lasted 20–45 minutes.

Making follow-up visits was not a problem for most patients, although a few reported lack of provider availability. Only a few patients remembered receiving reminder calls before an appointment. If they needed to talk with a provider between appointments, most patients were able to reach the provider or a nurse, but, again, some complained about the difficulty of reaching someone in the office or getting a response to messages.

Payments for Care

Over half of the patients had private insurance, with a co-payment ranging from 20 percent to 30 percent. Some supplemented their Medicare coverage with private insurance; only a few paid for their visits out of pocket or were covered solely by Medicare. Many of the patients did not find the fees burdensome, but some reported having to discontinue or limit their care at the center.

IM Center Director

The characteristics required of the director changed considerably over the course of the implementation. Originally, the ideal candidate was to be well-known in the field, be an outstanding academic, have a large patient base to bring to the hospital, and be an excellent educator. Unfortunately, few individuals have all these qualifications. The initial plan was to recruit a local practitioner who was already at the hospital (a biomedical-trained physician) and who had a successful CAM practice. The assumption was that he would bring that practice and those patents into the hospital-based center.

When that attempt failed, the board hired an acupuncturist who had also recently completed a biomedical degree. However, when the model he developed was rejected, he left the institution.

The director eventually chosen was a biomedical physician in internal medicine and an expert in CAM, particularly herbal therapies. Although she was well-known in the CAM community, she was not a high-profile person.

> It didn't evolve in the type of program that [was] envisioned. And part of it was the medical center, part of it was leadership in the program, and part of it was [making] compromises in order to get things done expediently. And the compromises were accepting the insurance issues, accepting substandard quarters, accepting

the concept of a physician-friendly model to begin with. Another compromise was in the leadership issue, because we needed some-body in that slot. [And] the number of individuals out there who could fill that slot was very limited. [We] sort of knew the [direc-tor] was going to be a bit of a compromise, even though [her] credentials were good. [Administrator P6]

The skill sets the director was expected to possess for this posi-tion were beyond most people's capabilities or the expectations of most CAM/IM centers. The director was from outside the hospital, so she did not have the background and cultural knowledge to function suc-cessfully as an administrator in the hospital bureaucracy. She faced the difficult task of coming in as an outsider without all the skills and understanding of organizational, cultural, and social norms neces-sary to successfully set up and run a clinic, especially a clinic that was attempting to integrate a nonbiomedical approach to medicine.

The hospital is also an academic institution, so the director was expected to conduct research and direct others in research. Although she had some success in the research component, this was not within the scope of her experience. The research expectations proved to be unrealistic given all the other tasks of the position, the biomedical bar-riers to CAM research (e.g., FDA, IND), and the pressure to write large grant applications without support or a track record.

Summary

Perhaps the greatest irony of this center's failure is that one of the key factors that contributed to its demise was the unanticipated effect of incorporation.

They made a huge mistake in the beginning. They set it up as a separate company, because they were afraid of a backlash . . . and this was a way for certain individuals to separate themselves . . . to protect themselves from the backlash. But there was no backlash. [Administrator P32]

In closing, it appears that multilevel legal constraints, as well as financial and practice-level incentives, drove the decision to establish the IM center as a professional corporation. The hospital also may be very risk-averse because of its structure and reputation. However, because the decisionmakers did not anticipate the significant financial obligations incorporation would entail, their attempt to deal with legal constraints and create a protective and lucrative corporate entity may have been the most significant barrier to their success.

> I suspect that we could have looked down the line and seen some of the practical clinical implications, bylaw implications, and so forth, to anything around this topic. [Administrator P12]

With regard to the patients, our key findings mirror previous research. The primary driving forces in patients seeking IM/CAM care are an increasingly consumerist approach to health care (i.e., patients want choices) and a desire for alternatives to pharmaceutical or surgical approaches to healing and health. From these perspectives, the shift in orientation is not simply about avoiding side effects or invasive procedures. Rather, it reflects a broader social shift in medical authority, a move away from a top-down biomedical hegemony and toward a more personally proactive attitude of individual responsibility for health and healing. This preference for an interactive approach to health and health care rests on a holistic perspective that incorporates the physical, mental, and spiritual dimensions of a patient's life. The patients in our sample wanted a knowledgeable physician with an inclusive medical armamentarium who could, as appropriate, draw on various medical models to facilitate their health and healing. These data underscore that patients want someone who takes the time to listen to them, communicate with them, and actively involve them in their own health care. The prestige of the institution did not appear to play a significant role in patients' use of the IM center; and what kept them coming back and referring others was strong personal relations with particular physicians and providers.

CHAPTER SEVEN

Conclusions: Facilitators and Barriers

The distinction is blurred between facilitators of and barriers to the center's success. Over the evolution of the IM center, factors that helped make it an attractive concept ultimately hindered its sustainability. To appreciate this paradox, we summarize the facilitators and barriers.

Facilitators of Integration

Some factors clearly worked in favor of the IM center. The first was the perception of strong support from the board of directors, although support was, in fact, limited. The sense that the program was a board initiative heightened its acceptability in the hospital community. A second factor that aided success was the hospital's reputation. Another attractive characteristic was its location, because all the referral services were in one organization. The fact that the IM center was initiated by the chief of medicine also had a significant impact.

> That's another reason I use [the IM center], because at least I know who these people are. I know it's not voodoo medicine. I know I can call them anytime, and vice versa. I'll actually end up paging them. They bend over backwards to try and accommodate. [Hospital Provider P46]

From a business perspective—at least during the planning phase—many factors could be considered facilitators. There was evidence, albeit misinterpreted, from the Eisenberg studies and others of large consumer demand for CAM and of patient willingness to pay out of pocket for these services. CAM appeared to be an untapped revenue source.

The hospital was responsive to this consumer demand. Within the institution, there was significant top-down support from two highly visible internal proponents and key members of the board of directors. This confluence resulted in the formation of a multidisciplinary task force and the development of a business plan. Both the board and the Medical Executive Committee approved the plan to implement a research-based CAM program.

An organizational home was found for the IM center in the hospital foundation. A professional corporation (PC) model was implemented to avoid unnecessary regulatory oversight, increase autonomy, avoid hospital salary caps, and provide incentives for patient volume through bonuses.

The ethos of the hospital made it a strong candidate for the IM program. It had a reputation and a track record of initiating innovative programs and meeting community needs, and it was a fairly entrepreneurial organization. In-house grand rounds and presentations provided a platform for promoting the center.

By setting up the center as a consultative practice, the developers ensured that it would not pose an economic threat to other hospital programs. Because the faculty were salaried, IM practitioners and physicians did not compete with them, although they did compete with the contract physicians. The IM center providers were perceived as specialists, which decreased the perceived threat.

The original design made a commitment to evidence-based practice and efficacy research. Evidence-based medicine was perceived as a marketing tool to increase CAM's acceptance. The fact that the key players in the center were western-trained biomedical doctors (internal medicine) helped allay biomedicine providers' fears about "voodoo medicine."

The implementation of a hospital-wide credentialing procedure that included hospital privileges was a major accomplishment that allowed the appointment of CAM providers.

Barriers to Integration

The center was perceived as a potential cash cow, but it was established at an inauspicious time because of the economic downturn in the health field. The business plan included unrealistic expectations and financial projections, and there was no strategic plan, vision, or operating budget. Marketing research was inadequate, and the predicted niche market turned out not to be viable.

The PC ultimately became an enormous barrier. It generated inflated provider salaries, high overhead for rent, and costly malpractice and director insurance, and it saddled the center with hospital billing costs for a moribund billing service.

The center's location, design, and décor also militated against its success. It was not the health spa setting that many CAM providers offered, nor was it an integral part of the hospital. It lacked adequate space to guarantee patient privacy. It was not "prestige space" and was located in an area where many competitors provided CAM treatments.

As for marketing, no plan was developed and no funds were made available for this critical business component, and hospital policy prevented the center from advertising in places likely to generate patients from the community.

Although initially planned as a cash clinic, the center was obliged to take the insurance provided for hospital employees as well as Medicare and Medi-Cal. This had a drastic impact on its ability to generate a profit. Adding to this reimbursement issue was the decision that all supplements and herbs would be sold by the hospital pharmacy rather than by the center, thus eliminating a major potential for profit. But even if the center had been profitable, the PC structure would have prevented the flow of revenue back to the hospital.

The institutional culture also posed barriers. Although there was not much overt opposition, widespread skepticism within the hospital did not help in generating a broad-based referral of patients. The referral issue was compounded because many departments had their own CAM therapies in place. And the perception of the clinic as a board-driven, top-down program increased resistance among staff who might have been referral sources. But the fear of a backlash from the medical staff had more impact than any actual backlash, because it forced the center staff into a defensive mode. They went to considerable lengths to assure hospital providers that they would not indulge in patient stealing.

The institution's prestigious reputation also made the medical staff wary about bringing in CAM modalities. Many believed that the center was a threat to their credibility. The lack of medical staff buy-in became important when the center was facing closure and could not elicit support from the medical staff or the board of directors.

The PC structure, which gave the center regulatory freedom and independence from oversight, also made it impossible to shift costs or bury losses, as it might have been able to do if it had been a department in the hospital. It was caught in a catch-22: to survive, it needed to increase its patient volume, but to attract patients it needed more staff and more space, both of which had become key targets in cutting costs.

The time frame allotted for the center's success was insufficient. Although it received seed money, a longer period of funding might have made it successful. We say "might," because—given all the other barriers—increased funding may simply have prolonged the agony.

Numerous barriers existed to the research center aspect of the plan. The center lacked the infrastructure to support junior researchers or planned outcomes studies, and it did not provide mentors. None of the staff were seasoned researchers with successful track records for grant awards. Further, the clinical and education demands were high, leaving little time for research. Center staff were also caught in a cumbersome administrative process to get IRB approval and to secure FDA IND applications for herb studies.

One of the barriers to research was that the institution was not set up for large outpatient clinics. On paper, the center was part of the foundation, but its status was administratively confusing to both center staff and hospital administrators.

On a cultural level, many CAM providers the director wanted to hire lacked appropriate licensure, and many of those who did work at the center were not conversant with hospital protocols and the referral process. They did not share the same norms as the medical staff, who had received their training within these systems. Hospital physicians worried that the center would not respect the protocol about returning referred patients—that if they sent patients to the center, they would not get them back. In many ways there was a clash of cultures—the two worlds that the center tried to integrate have different philosophies about illness and health care, different models of disease etiology, different languages, and different values.

Conclusion

Given all the barriers identified in this report, it is not surprising that the IM center did not survive. It was a high-risk venture that pursued a high-risk strategy. The risks may not have been obvious to the planners at the time, but in retrospect, the center was expected to do too much, too fast. In addition to becoming financially viable in a short time, it was expected to establish and sustain education and research components. These goals may have been overly ambitious, especially as this was the first integration program at the hospital.

What is surprising, though, is what the center's creators and participants did achieve. They managed to take a vision, create an IM center in a highly bureaucratic (and somewhat skeptical) environment, hire CAM providers, open for business, develop a clientele, and provide services with which clients were, for the most part, satisfied. The center and its outreach efforts promoted the integration of CAM and biomedicine, and various CAM modalities are being practiced in this institution today.

The full impact of the IM center may only become apparent in years to come. By thinking outside the box, the creators dared to merge CAM and biomedicine under the same roof. Their example has already inspired two center staff members from this story to establish IM centers elsewhere, and more attempts will no doubt follow.

In this case study, the word "success" can be applied in two ways: survival and impact. In terms of survival the center was not successful, but in terms of its impact, it can be considered successful.

Lessons for Future Centers

This bold experiment in integrative medicine offers some salutary lessons for any institution contemplating establishing a similar venture. While resolving these problems may not necessarily lead to a center's success, the probability of failure would be greatly reduced.

Vision

The starting point is to establish a vision. As we have noted in this study, different visions lead to different models of IM that have unique implications and outcomes. The vision should be clearly articulated, made public, and shared by the major stakeholders. This IM center suffered from the lack of a clear vision; the vision for it changed over time and was not widely shared. In addition, the vision should be expressed in a mission statement. Unless the major stakeholders are on the same page with regard to the mission/vision, it is unlikely that an IM center will succeed. The vision/mission should harmonize with the broader mission of the institution. Does it make sense for this institution to undertake this venture? What will the institution bring to the project that will make it unique or, at the very least, a center of quality?

Part of the process of creating a vision includes examining the philosophical elements of integrative medicine. IM subscribes to a different paradigm of illness, treatment, and care than biomedicine, which gives rise to a different set of health practices and a different view of health and health care. Are these beliefs compatible with the beliefs held in the institution? Can they be made compatible? Can they coexist without confusing the patients and causing conflict among the staff? To the extent that IM involves bringing CAM providers into the institution, it will be integrating a vitalistic paradigm with a materialistic one—biomedicine. These are very significant philosophical paradigm differences.

Market

Does a market exist for such a center in this institution? In this case study, the initiators established that a market for IM existed in the community, but they did not establish whether that would translate into market share for this center. While a center may make a contribution that is not market-driven (such as providing a valued service that contributes to the retention of a client base), this will entail quite different strategic decisions in the planning phase. If the center is expected to make a profit or at least recover its costs, market research is crucial. No matter how prestigious the institution, if you build it, they will not necessarily come.

Advocates

Strong advocates are necessary to launch a program within an institution. Advocates must be credible and powerful. They may not have to do much actual promoting, but the perception that they are advocating for the program can be a powerful incentive for others to join the project or, at the very least, not work against it. The need for advocates occurs at many levels in an institution's hierarchy and may change at different points of the process. In this institution, the support of the board and administrative/medical staff leaders ensured that the program got started.

Business Plan and Finances

The key requirement is not just to have a business plan but to have a *realistic* business plan. The plan should be tied to two important criteria: a specific market assessment of the potential clientele and a full assessment of all costs that will be associated with the start-up. The time frame in which the center is expected to become self-sustaining must also be realistic. In this study, no center could have been profitable in the time frame allowed, given the costs and the lack of a clientele. Planners must carefully examine the assumptions on which any business plan is based, and the business plan must be flexible. Circumstances change, and the business plan should also change. In this case study, not only was the business plan unrealistic, it lagged behind what was actually happening—by the time it was changed, the deficit was enough to bring an end to the clinic. Part of the business plan must focus on what services can be billed to insurance companies and what type of practitioners can bill for them. Start-up funds are a crucial part of financing and must be in place for a sufficient period to allow the center to survive. Many IM centers have been established through philanthropy.

Legal Matters

The establishment of an IM center raises numerous legal issues. Credentialing providers and ensuring that they are covered by malpractice insurance can be extremely complicated. In this case, determining the legal entity under which the clinic would operate proved to be the most important decision made by its planners. The legal possibilities will help shape the IM center and may lead to changes in the vision.

Strategy

Until all these issues are resolved, it would be premature to design or construct a center. The resolution of the issues will dictate the implementation of the center. A center that is constructed for a nonexistent clientele is unlikely to survive. It is difficult to envision a center with a broad range of CAM practitioners if they cannot legally practice in the institution, cannot be covered by malpractice insurance, and cannot bill for their services under existing insurance.

Assuming that all the issues have been hammered out, strategic decisions revolve around the following:

1. What model of IM is to be implemented? A distributive model spread throughout the institution? A consultative model, in which patients are referred for consults but returned to the division from which they came? A stand-alone clinic offering primary care? A specialty clinic? A virtual clinic? Each of these options poses different challenges and requires quite different strategic decisions.

2. Will it be a treatment clinic, a research institute, an educational program, or some combination of these?

3. Will it be therapy-based (e.g., mind-body therapy, herbal therapies); disease-based (e.g., chronic illness); adjunctive therapy (e.g., for cancer patients); focused on symptoms (e.g., pain clinic); or some combination of these?

4. What professions, practices, and providers will be appointed? Will western-trained biomedical providers provide oversight and be the dominant profession in the center?
5. Who will be the clients? The "worried well" who have resources? Underserved populations? Persons who are already patients in the institution? A whole new population?

Once these questions have been answered, much of what follows is logistics and promotion. How do you persuade others in the institution that such a program is a legitimate and viable exercise? What will be the IM center's institutional home? What department or program will it be part of? Where will it be located physically? What will the physical structure look like? How will hospital staff be encouraged to use the center? How will the patient base be built and retained? What kind of marketing will be required? How important will referrals be, and how can they be ensured?

Next, the question arises of who should direct the center. Until the type of clinic has been outlined and potential challenges identified, it is difficult to specify the skill set that will be important for a director. One person is unlikely to have all the necessary skills and experience. More than one person may be appointed to carry out different functions of the program. For example, many institutions separate clinical, research, and educational tasks.

Although this IM center failed to sustain itself, the lessons learned can help the next generation of centers for integrative medicine achieve success.

Expert Panel

Twelve persons were invited to participate in a one-day workshop at RAND to join the project staff in a discussion of the findings of this study. The panel participants were chosen because of their expertise in integrative medicine. Some had designed, implemented, and run programs, and some had conducted IM research. Although the results of this workshop are not included in the case study report, they had a major influence on the study by providing strong evidence that this situation was not unique. For the most part, the expert panel recognized the events at the IM center as being quite common in centers of this kind. They also provided a strong counterbalance to the conclusion that could have been drawn—that the IM center was an unsuccessful experiment. By sharing their experience and knowledge, they enabled us to place this story in a broader context. The panel's insightful feedback made clear that we had witnessed the early evolution in the construction of a center for integrative medicine in a hospital setting. The institution in this case study was not the first to attempt this challenge (in fact, the hospital task force visited several other sites), but it was in the first wave.

Methods

We told the story of the center in "acts" and solicited feedback periodically. This approach allowed us to identify holes in the story where the panel could not follow our account and allowed the panel participants to make comparisons with other centers around core themes. The story was presented in four acts: Act I, The Beginning; Act II, The End of the Beginning; Act III, The Beginning of the End; and Act IV, Devolution. For each act we presented the panel with a set of questions to encourage discussion.

Act I

1. What role has the board played elsewhere?
2. How important have internal advocates been?
3. How important has a business plan been?
4. How important has agreement been over what IM is?

Act II

1. Has the professional corporation model been used elsewhere?
2. Can a clinic survive on third-party payers?
3. Could such a model succeed?
4. Is the external CAM/IM community a realistic source for patients?
5. Do networks develop around IM?

Act III

1. How similar is this story to other IM center stories?
2. How many of these problems could have been avoided?
3. Is a hospital an appropriate setting for IM?
4. If so, what model has the best chance of success?

Results

The Board

The expert panel agreed that support from the institutional board of directors is important, but the role of the board can vary considerably. For some centers, it is essential. The board can provide strong leadership; play an advisory role (not policy-oriented); help decide what to do; provide input into the business plan and bylaws; and provide fundraising. But the board serves different functions at different times. It is important that the governance board help the program fit the needs of the institution. Furthermore, the board can give credibility to the center. Board buy-in was thought to be important for policy, fundraising, and fiscal control. The board's role should be explicit; it should be a stabilizing force and should provide links back into the larger institution.

Advocates

The expert panel believed that internal advocates are key—a necessary but not sufficient condition for success. The major internal advocates' role is not time-dependent. A center needs advocates at all levels in the institution. In this case, the planners attempted to alter the orthodox community, but they did not get the "planets aligned" at all levels: the board, the key internal institutional players, and those in the field. A successful program must have advocates at all three levels.

The Model

The panel noted that center developers often encounter "huge model confusion" and have difficulty operationalizing a vision. They may have to change the model numerous times. The models used by other institutions have been very dynamic and continue to be in flux several years into the operation of the new centers. For example, patients may want primary care, but the center may be set up as a collaborative-consultative model.

The Business Plan

The panel participants said the business plan used in this case study was "a very familiar one." Process literature did not exist to design a business model for this type of clinic at that time, and there was a lack of concrete data on which to build a plan. Understandably, this lack of information resulted in a totally unrealistic business plan. Many IM centers have business plans that are continuously changing. A business plan, the panel agreed, is important for launching a program, for board buy-in, and as an analytical device, as it forces an accounting of many important details. However, the plan must be dynamic and capable of responding to challenges that arise. In the case study, the IM group was locked into a rigid legal model/business plan and could not adapt or be flexible.

Some panel members suggested that the strong board support and the internal advocates might have interfered with performing "due diligence" in the business planning stage. The power of an important individual's advocacy can be very persuasive, and enthusiasm can lead to poor judgment. Likewise, the powerful perception of board support can allow a poorly designed business plan to escape scrutiny.

The panel members questioned the manner in which the results of Eisenberg's surveys were interpreted. If the data on CAM users include self-care, the actual potential for provider-based care is much lower than the numbers touted in the surveys. Furthermore, if you compare the amount of money Eisenberg cited as being spent on CAM care with overall health care spending in the United States, the CAM spending is "a drop in the bucket."

The panel believed that the planners' focus on money was naïve; however, these were the early days of IM groups, before "the landscape was littered with failures." The panel was strong in its opinion that the decision to accept insurance sounded the first "death knell" for the center. The cash-and-carry model would have been more financially viable.

The Professional Corporation

The decision to set up the center as a professional corporation was a fatal flaw, in the opinion of the panel. It was also seen as the most surprising decision. However, research shows that the higher the legal liability for medical groups, the higher the quality of care. Liability provides the incentive to select the right (and most competent) CAM practitioners. If physicians are liable for bad referrals, they will not make them. In that sense, there was at least some justification for choosing the corporate model.

Leadership

The panel perceived a mismatch between the skills needed in a director and the talents of the person who was selected. They thought a very structured job description should have been used to guide the search process. But the panel acknowledged that few people qualified for the position at that time. One option might have been to hold off another year.

Turf Tension Between Primary Care and the Consultative Model

The panel noted that all IM clinics deal with the issue of turf tension. In a sense, "consultative care" is viewed as a Trojan horse, because IM is holistic and by nature focuses on primary care. Patients illustrate this problem every day, because some want their IM providers to be their primary care providers. Also, many MDs do not want to be on call for this particular patient population. Thus, the model can morph from consultative care to primary care. In some cases, the IM group's ability to work with "shipwreck" patients endears it to outside MDs. These clinics actually get referrals because they offer primary care for patients whose biomedical doctors have run out of options for them.

Clinic/Outcomes Research

Several panelists discussed the assumption that a clinic can easily provide research. They said that the patient population tends to be too heterogeneous to supply the power to find effects. The only way such research would have validity would be if a clinic were run as a research lab and did not provide the usual patient care.

Referrals

The panel made an interesting case that unless you have a denominator of how many referrals are possible, it is difficult to determine whether MD referrals are good or bad at any center. A denominator might be created by picking several diseases known to be treated with CAM (e.g., fibromyalgia) and tracing back the number of likely referrals. In this clinic, the IM group did not focus on cultivating the largest source of referrals (patient and self-referrals). This was a big mistake. Patients could self-refer, but the location was suboptimal for some patients. Patients are mixed in the way they rate putting CAM into the hospital setting. In other clinics, about half the patients liked the credibility delivered by the clinic's location in a teaching hospital (because they felt "safe"), while the other half found it inconvenient.

In other such clinics, most of the MD referrals come from subspecialties; IM groups can cultivate these physicians by serving on department committees and developing relationships with them. Lecturing may not be the best way to do this.

However, this IM center may simply not have operated long enough to generate MD referrals. Some panel members thought the center did not function long enough for a network approach to succeed for CAM providers.

Summary

The panel's main conclusions were that the attempt to create an IM center in a hospital was courageous in that the hospital took the first step in the evolutionary process. Therefore, this attempt should not be viewed as a catastrophic failure. The participants believed that the program failed because the institution did not provide the necessary political and financial backing required for longevity. The center never had the chance to be successful. A viable center takes more than 2.5 years to grow. The panel noted that even "turbocharged" programs are typically in the red for three to four years. The panel noted that it was not reasonable to expect all three prongs of the IM model (the clinical, research, and education components) to be viable in such a short time.

The panel highlighted the risk-aversion issues that ran as a "reactionary thread" through the entire story. Risk-aversion is counter to innovation, and fear can trump vision. As one panel member said, "You should listen to the lawyers, but you shouldn't let them drive the business model." It seemed to this panel that the lawyers drove the center into the PC model to avoid risk; however, in doing so, they voided the vision of those who had developed the model.

The lessons from the case study can be applied as a blueprint for the issues and dangers that occur in creating IM centers. In answer to our questions, the panel reached the following conclusions:

How similar was this story to their experiences? The issues were not unique to the case study.

How avoidable was the outcome? The PC structure could have been avoided. The PC model led to a "cascade of problems" that undermined the center.

Is the hospital an appropriate environment for IM? Because of the PC structure, the case study did not answer this question. The relationship with the hospital was "murky."

Was there a market for this center? There was a market, but the program erred in accepting all types of patients and trying to be all things to all people. By not defining and then focusing on a homogeneous group—such as high utilizers—the center was set up to fail. The center lacked an identity that could have been used to brand it and market it to patients, third-party payers, and foundations/philanthropists.

How valid was the assumption that patient demand was not already being met? The panel agreed that the hospital did not know the answer to this question, and probably still does not know.

Hospital-Based Integrative Medicine Expert Panel
RAND Corporation, Santa Monica, CA
Monday, April 24, 2006

John A. Astin, PhD
California Pacific Medical Center
San Francisco, CA

Jeanne A. Drisko, MD
Hugh D Riordan Professor of Orthomolecular Medicine
Director, Program in Integrative Medicine
Member, Kansas Cancer Research Institute
University of Kansas Medical Center
Kansas City, KS

David M. Eisenberg, MD
Director, Division for Research and
Education in Complementary and
Integrative Medical Therapies
Osher Institute at Harvard Medical School
Boston, MA

Barbara Findlay, R.N., B.S.N.
Vice President
Samueli Institute
Alexandria, VA

Susan Folkman, PhD
Osher Foundation Distinguished Professor of Integrative Medicine, UCSF
Member, UCSF Comprehensive Cancer Center
Director, UCSF Osher Center
University of California, San Francisco
San Francisco, CA

Wayne B. Jonas, M.D.
President and CEO
Samueli Institute
Alexandria, VA

William Lafferty, MD
Director, Health & Policy Research Track
University of Washington
Seattle, WA

John Longhurst, M.D., Ph.D.
Professor of Medicine,
Susan Samueli Center for Integrative Medicine
Professor and Associate Dean for Programs and Development, UCI College
of Medicine
Irvine, CA

Kenneth R. Pelletier, PhD, MD(hc)
Clinical Professor of Medicine
Director, Corporate Health Improvement Program (CHIP)
Department of Medicine
University of Arizona School of Medicine and the University of California School of Medicine (UCSF)

LTC Richard Petri, Jr., MC
Director, Center for Integrative Medicine
William Beaumont Army Medical Center
El Paso, TX

Jay Udani, MD, CPI (IM)
Medical Director, Integrative Medicine Program
Northridge Hospital
Assistant Clinical Professor at the UCLA / Geffen School of Medicine
Northridge, CA

Sara Warber, M.D.
Co-Director,
University of Michigan Integrative Medicine
Assistant Professor,
Department of Family Medicine
Ann Arbor, MI

RAND *MG591-letterA.2*

Brief Time Line

Table B.1
Brief Time Line

IM Center Time Line	1996	June-97	May-98	August-98	May-00	July-01
Medical director investigates CAM for hospital	▓					
Task force formed; site visits take place	▓					
Complementary medicine program business plan presented to board		▓				
IM center final director hired			▓			
IM center up and running, doors open to patients				▓		
Hospital administrator joins to "stop the bleeding"					▓	
IM center folded into a department in the hospital						▓

References

Astin, John A., "Why patients use alternative medicine: results of a national study," *JAMA*, Vol. 279, No. 19, May 20, 1998, pp. 1548–1553.

Astin, John A., Ariane Marie, Kenneth R. Pelletier, Erik Hansen, and William L. Haskell, "A review of the incorporation of complementary and alternative medicine by mainstream physicians," in P. B. Fontanarosa, ed., *Alternative Medicine: An Objective Assessment*, American Medical Association, 2000.

Barnes, Patricia M., Eve Powell-Griner, Kim McFann, and Richard L. Nahin, "Complementary and alternative medicine use among adults: United States, 2002," *Advance Data*, No. 343, May 27, 2004, pp. 1–19.

Barrett, Bruce, "Alternative, complementary, and conventional medicine: Is integration upon us?" *Journal of Alternative and Complementary Medicine*, Vol. 9, No. 3, Jun 2003, pp. 417–427.

Becker, Howard, "Problems of inference and proof in participant observation," *American Sociological Review*, Vol. 26, No. 6, 1958, pp. 652–660.

Berman, Brian M., B. Krishna Singh, Lixing Lao, Betsy B. Singh, Kevin S. Ferentz, and Susan M. Hartnoll, "Physicians' attitudes toward complementary or alternative medicine: A regional survey," *J Am Board Fam Pract*, Vol. 8, No. 5, Sep-Oct 1995, pp. 361–366.

Bernard, H. Russell, *Research methods in anthropology: Qualitative and quantitative approaches*, 4th Edition, Lanham, MD: AltaMira Press, 2006.

Bhattacharya, Bhaswati, "M.D. programs in the United States with complementary and alternative medicine education: An ongoing listing," *Journal of Alternative and Complementary Medicine*, Vol. 4, No. 3, Fall 1998, pp. 325–335.

Bhattacharya, Bhaswati, "M.D. programs in the United States with complementary and alternative medicine education opportunities: An ongoing listing," *Journal of Alternative and Complementary Medicine*, Vol. 6, No. 1, Feb 2000, pp. 77–90.

Blanchet, K. D., "University Center for Complementary and Alternative Medicine at Stony Brook," *Journal of Alternative and Complementary Therapies*, Vol. 4, 1998, pp. 327–332.

Borkan, J., J. Neher, O. Anson, and B. Smoker, "Referrals for alternative therapies," *The Journal of Family Practice*, Vol. 39, No. 6, 1994, pp. 545–550.

Caronna, Carol A., Seth S. Pollack, and W. Richard Scott, *Cases and contexts: Investigating micro-macro linkages through an embedded case study design*, unpublished RAND research, 1997.

Coates, J. R., and Kim A. Jobst, "Integrated healthcare: A way forward for the next five years? A discussion document from the Prince of Wales's Initiative on Integrated Medicine," *Journal of Alternative and Complementary Medicine*, Vol. 4, No. 2, Summer 1998, pp. 209–247.

Cohen, Marc M., "CAM practitioners and 'regular' doctors: Is integration possible?" *The Medical Journal of Australia*, Vol. 180, No. 12, Jun 21, 2004, pp. 645–646.

Coulter, Ian D., Ron D. Hays, and C. D. Danielson, "The Chiropractic Satisfaction Questionnaire," *Topics in Clinical Chiropractic*, Vol. 1, 1994, pp. 40–43.

Coulter, Ian D., *Chiropractic: A Philosophy for Alternative Health Care*, Oxford: Butterworth-Heineman, 1999.

Coulter, Ian, "Integration and Paradigm Clash," in Tovey, P., Easthope, G., and Adams, J., eds., *The Mainstreaming of Complementary and Alternative Medicine: Studies in Social Context*, London and New York: Routledge Taylor & Francis Group, 2004, pp. 103–122.

Coulter, Ian D., and Evan M. Willis, "The rise and rise of complementary and alternative medicine: a sociological perspective," *The Medical Journal of Australia*, Vol. 180, No. 11, Jun 7, 2004, pp. 587-589.

Dalen, James E., "'Conventional' and 'unconventional' medicine: Can they be integrated?" *Archives of Internal Medicine*, Vol. 158, No. 20, Nov 9, 1998, pp. 2179–2181.

Daly, Deborah, "Alternative medicine courses taught at U.S. medical schools: An ongoing list," *Journal of Alternative and Complementary Medicine*, Vol. 1, No. 2, Summer 1995, pp. 205–207.

Daly, Deborah, "Alternative medicine courses taught at U.S. medical schools: An ongoing list," *Journal of Alternative and Complementary Medicine*, Vol. 3, No. 4, Winter 1997, pp. 405–410.

de Vries, Hein, Wies Weijts, Margo Dijkstra, and Gerjo Kok, "The utilization of qualitative and quantitative data for Health Education Program planning, implementation, and evaluation: A spiral approach," *Health Education & Behavior*, Vol. 19, 1992, pp. 101–115.

Druss, Benjamin G., and Robert A. Rosenheck, "Association between use of unconventional therapies and conventional medical services," *JAMA*, Vol. 282, No. 7, Aug 18, 1999, pp. 651–656.

Edgerton, Robert B., and Lewis L. Langness, *Methods and styles in the study of culture*, San Francisco: Chandler & Sharp Publishers, 1974.

Eisenberg, David M., Ted J. Kaptchuk, and Debi Arcarese, *Alternative Medicine: Implications for Clinical Practice and Research*, Boston, MA: Harvard Medical School, Dept. Medicine Elective ME549. J121, Office of Educational Development, 1993.

Eisenberg, David M., R. C. Kessler, Cindy Foster, Frances E. Norlock, David R. Calkins, and Thomas L. Delbanco, "Unconventional medicine in the United States. Prevalence, costs, and patterns of use," *New England Journal of Medicine*, Vol. 328, No. 4, 1993, pp. 246–252.

Eisenberg, David M., Roger B. Davis, Susan L. Ettner, Scott Appel, Sonja A. Wilkey, Maria I. Van Rompay, and Ronald C. Kessler, "Trends in alternative medicine use in the United States, 1990–1997: Results of a follow-up national survey," *JAMA*, Vol. 280, No. 18, Nov 11, 1998, pp. 1569–1575.

Eisenberg, David M., Ronald C. Kessler, Maria I. Van Rompay, Ted J. Kaptchuk, Sonja A. Wilkey, Scott Appel, and Roger B. Davis, "Perceptions about complementary therapies relative to conventional therapies among adults who use both: Results from a national survey," *Annals of Internal Medicine*, Vol. 135, No. 5, Sep 4, 2001, pp. 344–351.

Eisenberg, David M., "David M. Eisenberg, MD: Integrative medicine research pioneer. Interview by Karolyn A Gazella and Suzanne Snyder," *Alternative Therapies in Health and Medicine*, Vol. 12, No. 1, Jan-Feb 2006, pp. 72–79.

Eisenberg, Merrill, and Nancy Swanson, "Organizational network analysis as a tool for program evaluation," *Evaluation & The Health Professions*, Vol. 19, No. 4, 1996, pp. 488–507.

Ernst, Edzard, Karl-Ludwig Resch, and Adrian R. White, "Complementary medicine. What physicians think of it: a meta-analysis," *Archives of Internal Medicine*, Vol. 155, No. 22, Dec 11–25, 1995, pp. 2405–2408.

Fielding, Nigel G., and Raymond M. Lee, *Using computers in qualitative research*, Newbury Park, CA: Sage Publications, 1991.

Fontanarosa, Phil B., and George D. Lundberg, "Complementary, Alternative, Unconventional, and Integrative Medicine: Call for Papers for the Annual Coordinated Theme Issues of the AMA Journals," *JAMA*, Vol. 278, No. 23, Dec 17, 1997, pp. 2111–2112.

Giddens, Anthony, *Runaway World: How Globalization is Reshaping Our Lives*, New York: Routledge, 2000.

Gilchrist, Valerie J., "Key Informant Interviews," in Benjamin F. Crabtree and William L. Miller, eds., *Doing qualitative research*, Newbury Park, CA: Sage Publications, 1992, pp. 70–89 (Chapter 74).

Glaser, Barney G., and Anselm Strauss, *The discovery of grounded theory: Strategies for qualitative research*, Chicago: Aldine, 1967.

Graham, Robert E., Andrew C. Ahn, Roger B. Davis, Bonnie B. O'Connor, David M. Eisenberg, and Russell S. Phillips, "Use of complementary and alternative medical therapies among racial and ethnic minority adults: Results from the 2002 National Health Interview Survey," *Journal of the National Medical Association*, Vol. 97, No. 4, Apr 2005, pp. 535–545.

Hengstberger-Sims, Cecily, and M. A. McMillan, "Stakeholder evaluation: A model for decision making in problem-based learning," *Nurse Education Today*, Vol. 11, No. 6, Dec 1991, pp. 439–447.

Hsiao, An-Fu, Ron D. Hays, Gery W. Ryan, Ian D. Coulter, Robert M. Andersen, Mary L. Hardy, David L. Diehl, Kit K. Hui, and Neil S. Wenger, "A self-report measure of clinicians' orientation toward integrative medicine," *Health Services Research*, Vol. 40, No. 5 (Part 1), 2005, pp. 1553–1569.

Hsiao, An-Fu, Gery W. Ryan, Ron D. Hays, Ian D. Coulter, Robert M. Andersen, and Neil S. Wenger, "Variations in provider conceptions of integrative medicine," *Social Science & Medicine*, Vol. 62, No. 12, Jun 2006, pp. 2973–2987.

Hyman, Mark A., "The real alternative medicine: reconsidering conventional medicine," *Alternative therapies in health and medicine*, Vol. 11, No. 5, Sep-Oct 2005, pp. 10–12.

Institute of Medicine (IOM), *Complementary and Alternative Medicine (CAM) in the United States*, Washington, DC: The National Academies Press, 2005.

Jacobs, Joseph J., "Building bridges between two worlds: the NIH's office of alternative medicine," *Academic Medicine*, Vol. 70, No. 1, Jan 1995, pp. 40–41.

Jinnett, Kimberly, Ian D. Coulter, and Paul Koegel, "Cases, contexts, and care: The need for grounded network analysis," *Social Networks and Health*, Vol. 8, 2002, pp. 101–110.

Johnson, Jeffrey C., *Selecting ethnographic informants*, Thousand Oaks, CA: Sage Publications, 1990.

Jonas, Wayne B., "Wayne B. Jonas, MD: supporting the scientific foundation of integrative medicine. Interviewed by Karolyn A. Gazella and Suzanne Snyder," *Alternative therapies in health and medicine*, Vol. 11, No. 5, Sep-Oct 2005, pp. 68–74.

Kaptchuk, Ted J., and Franklin G. Miller, "Viewpoint: what is the best and most ethical model for the relationship between mainstream and alternative medicine: opposition, integration, or pluralism?" *Academic Medicine*, Vol. 80, No. 3, Mar 2005, pp. 286–290.

Kelner, Merrijoy, Oswald Hall, and Ian D. Coulter, "Chiropractors. Do They Help? A study of their education and practice," Toronto: Fitzhenry & Whiteside, 1980.

Kim, Catherine, and Yeong S. Kwok, "Navajo use of native healers," *Archives of Internal Medicine*, Vol. 158, No. 20, Nov 9, 1998, pp. 2245–2249.

Larson, Laurie, "Integrating integrative medicine—a how-to guide," *Trustee*, Vol. 58, No. 10, Nov-Dec 2005, pp. 11, 14–16, 21–22.

Lincoln, Yvonna S., and Egon G. Guba, *Naturalistic inquiry*, Newbury Park, CA: Sage Publications, 1985.

McGregor, Katherine J., and Edmund R. Peay, "The choice of alternative therapy for health care: Testing some propositions," *Social Science & Medicine*, Vol. 43, No. 9, Nov 1996, pp. 1317–1327.

Mead, Nicola, and Peter Bower, "Patient-centredness: A conceptual framework and review of the empirical literature," *Social Science & Medicine*, Vol. 51, No. 7, Oct 2000, pp. 1087–1110.

Micozzi, Marc S., "Culture, anthropology, and the return of 'complementary medicine,'" *Medical Anthropology Quarterly*, Vol. 16, No. 4, Dec 2002, pp. 398–403.

Miles, Matthew B., and A. Michael Huberman, *Qualitative Data Analysis: An expanded sourcebook*, Thousand Oaks, CA: Sage Publications, 1994.

Miller, William L., and Benjamin F. Crabtree, "Primary care research: A multimethod typology and qualitative road map," in Benjamin F. Crabtree and William L. Miller, eds., *Qualitative Research: Research Methods for Primary Care*, London: Sage Publications, 1992.

Monson, Nancy, "Alternative Medicine Education at Medical Schools: Are They Catching On?" *Alternative & Complementary Therapies*, April/May 1995, pp. 168–170.

Moore, N. G., "Psychiatry and alternative medicine: constructing a rationale for integration," *Alternative Therapies in Health and Medicine*, Vol. 3, No. 2, Mar 1997, pp. 24, 26–27, 114 passim.

Morrissey, Joseph P., Mark Tausig, and Michael L. Lindsey, *Network Analysis Methods for Mental Health Service System Research: A Comparison of Two Community Support Systems*, Washington, DC: National Institute of Mental Health, 1985.

Morrissey, Joseph P., Matthew C. Johnsen, and Michael O. Calloway, "Evaluating performance and change in mental health systems serving children and youth: an interorganizational network approach," *Journal of Mental Health Administration*, Vol. 24, No. 1, 1997, pp. 4–22.

Morse, Janice M., "Designing funded qualitative research," in Norman K. Denzin and Yvonna S. Lincoln, eds., *Handbook of Qualitative Research*, Thousand Oaks, CA: Sage Publications, 1994, pp. 220–235.

Muhr, Thomas, ATLAS.ti, The Knowledge Workbench Version 5.0 for Windows. Scientific Software Development. Copyright 1997– 2004.

Mullen, Patricia D., and R. Reynolds, "The potential of grounded theory for health education research: linking theory and practice," *Health Education Monographs*, Vol. 6, No. 3, Fall 1978, pp. 280–294.

Muscat, M., "Beth Israel's Center for Health and Healing: realizing the goal of fully integrative care," *Alternative Therapies in Health and Medicine*, Vol. 6, No. 5, Sep 2000, pp. 100–101.

National Center for Complementary and Alternative Medicine (NCCAM), "Expanding Horizons of Healthcare: Five-Year Strategic Plan, 2001-2005." As of May 29, 2007:
http://nccam.nih.gov/about/plans/fiveyear

Ni, Hanyu, Catherine Simile, and Ann M. Hardy, "Utilization of complementary and alternative medicine by United States adults: results from the 1999 national health interview survey," *Medical Care*, Vol. 40, No. 4, Apr 2002, pp. 353–358.

Paramore, L. Clark, "Use of alternative therapies: estimates from the 1994 Robert Wood Johnson Foundation National Access to Care Survey," *Journal of Pain and Symptom Management*, Vol. 13, No. 2, Feb 1997, pp. 83–89.

Patton, Michael Quinn, *Qualitative evaluation and research methods*, Newbury Park, CA: Sage Publications, 1990.

Pelletier, Kenneth R., John A. Astin, and William L. Haskell, "Current trends in the integration and reimbursement of complementary and alternative medicine by managed care organizations (MCOs) and insurance providers: 1998 update and cohort analysis," *American Journal of Health Promotion*, Vol. 14, No. 2, Nov-Dec 1999, pp. 125–133.

Pelletier, Kenneth R. and John A. Astin, "Integration and reimbursement of complementary and alternative medicine by managed care and insurance providers," *Alternative Therapies in Health and Medicine*, Vol. 8, No. 1, Jan-Feb 2002, pp. 38–39, 42, 44 passim.

Pfaffenberger, Bryan, *Microcomputer applications in qualitative research*, Newbury Park: Sage Publications, 1988.

Ranjan, R., "Magic or logic: Can 'alternative' medicine be scientifically integrated into modern medical practice?" *Advances in Mind-Body Medicine*, Vol. 14, 1998, pp. 43–73.

Ruggie, Mary, "Mainstreaming complementary therapies: new directions in health care," *Health Affairs (Project Hope)*, Vol. 24, No. 4, Jul-Aug 2005, pp. 980–990.

Ryan, Gery, and H. Russell Bernard, "Data management and analysis methods," in Norman Denzin and Yvonna Lincoln, eds., *Handbook of Qualitative Research, 2nd ed.*, Thousand Oaks, CA: Sage Publications, 2000, pp. 769–802.

SAS Institute Inc. SAS OnlineDoc® Version 8, for 1999.

Savage, Grant T., John D. Blair, Michael J. Benson, and Byron Hale, "Urban-rural hospital affiliations: Assessing control, fit, and stakeholder issues strategically," *Health Care Management Review*, Vol. 17, No. 1, Winter 1992, pp. 35–49.

Scott, John, *Social network analysis: A handbook*, London: Sage Publications, 1991.

Siahpush, Mohammad, "Postmodern values, dissatisfaction with conventional medicine, and popularity of alternative therapies," *Journal of Sociology*, Vol. 34, No. 1, Mar 1998, pp. 58–70.

Sirois, Fushia M., and Mary L. Gick, "An investigation of the health beliefs and motivations of complementary medicine clients," *Social Science & Medicine*, Vol. 55, No. 6, Sep 2002, pp. 1025–1037.

Spradley, James P., *The ethnographic interview*, New York: Holt, Rinehart, and Winston, 1979.

Tashakkori, Abbas, and Charles Teddlie, *Mixed Methodology: Combining Qualitative and Quantitative Approaches*, Thousand Oaks, CA: Sage Publications, 1998.

Ullman, Dana, "The mainstreaming of alternative medicine," *Healthcare Forum Journal*, Vol. 3, 1993, pp. 24–30.

University of Arizona. As of May 29, 2007:
http://integrativemedicine.arizona.edu/about2.html

U.S. Department of Health and Human Services, HHS News, HHS Issues Final Rule Addressing Physician Self-Referrals, January 3, 2001. As of May 29, 2007:
http://www.hhs.gov/news/press/2001pres/20010103.html

Van de Ven, Andrew H., "On the nature, formation, and maintenance of relations among organizations," *Academy of Management Review*, Vol. 1, October 1976, pp. 24–36.

Van de Ven, Andrew H., and Diane L. Ferry, *Measuring and Assessing Organizations*, New York: John Wiley, 1980.

Van Maanen, John, *Qualitative Methodology*, Beverly Hills, CA: Sage Publications, 1979.

Vohra, Sunita, Kymm Feldman, Brad Johnston, Kellie Waters, and Heather Boon, "Integrating complementary and alternative medicine into academic medical centers: experience and perceptions of nine leading centers in North America," *BMC Health Services Research*, Vol. 5, 2005, p. 78.

Wasserman, Stanley, and Katherine Faust, *Social Network Analysis: Methods and Applications*, New York: Cambridge University Press, 1994.

Weeks, John, "Major Trends in the Integration of Complementary and Alternative Medicine," in N. Faass, ed., *Integrating Complementary Medicine into Health Systems*, Gaithersburg, MD: Aspen, 2001, pp. 4–11.

Weil, Andrew, Editorial. "Integrative Medicine." 1998, Vol. 1, No. 1.

Weil, Andrew, Personal correspondence. Apr 2000.

Weiss, Carol H., "The stakeholder approach to evaluation: Origins and promise," in Ernest R. House, ed., *New Directions in Educational Evaluation*, London: Falmer Press, 1986.

Wetzel, Miriam S., David M. Eisenberg, and Ted J. Kaptchuk, "Courses involving complementary and alternative medicine at US medical schools," *JAMA*, Vol. 280, No. 9, Sep 2, 1998, pp. 784–787.

Wetzel, Miriam S., Ted J. Kaptchuk, Aviad Haramati, and David M. Eisenberg, "Complementary and alternative medical therapies: Implications for medical education," *Annals of Internal Medicine*, Vol. 138, No. 3, Feb 4, 2003, pp. 191–196.

White, Adrian R., A. Mitchell, and Edzard Ernst, "Familiarization with complementary medicine: Report of a new course for primary care physicians," *Journal of Alternative and Complementary Medicine*, Vol. 2, No. 2, 1996, pp. 307–314.

White, Adrian R., Karl-Ludwig Resch, and Edzard Ernst, "A survey of complementary practitioners' fees, practice, and attitudes to working within the National Health Service," *Complementary Therapies in Medicine*, Vol. 5, 1997, pp. 210–214.

Whitehead, Carlton J., John D. Blair, R. R. Smith, Timothy W. Nix, and Grant T. Savage, "Stakeholder supportiveness and strategic vulnerability: implications for competitive strategy in the HMO industry," *Health Care Management Review*, Vol. 14, No. 3, Summer 1989, pp. 65–76.

Widra, Linda S., and Myron D. Fottler, "Determinants of HMO success: The case of Complete Health," *Health Care Management Review*, Vol. 17, No. 2, Spring 1992, pp. 33–44.

Wiseman, Nigel, "Designations of Medicines," *Evidence-Based Complementary and Alternative Medicine*, Vol. 1, No. 3, Dec 2004, pp. 327–329.

Wolsko, Peter M., David M. Eisenberg, Roger B. Davis, and Russell S. Phillips, "Use of mind-body medical therapies," *Journal of General Internal Medicine*, Vol. 19, No. 1, Jan 2004, pp. 43–50.

Wootton, Jacqueline C., and Andrew Sparber, "Surveys of complementary and alternative medicine: Part IV. Use of alternative and complementary therapies for rheumatologic and other diseases," *Journal of Alternative and Complementary Medicine*, Vol. 7, No. 6, 2001, pp. 715–721.

Wright, Eric R., and I. Michael Shuff, "Specifying the integration of mental health and primary health care services for persons with HIV/AIDS: The Indiana integration of care project," *Social Networks*, Vol. 17, 1995, pp. 319–340.

Yin, Robert K., Peter G. Bateman, and Gwendolyn B. Moore, *Case Studies and Organizational Innovation: Strengthening the Connection*, Washington, DC: Cosmos, 1983.

Yin, Robert K., *Case study research: Design and methods*, Thousand Oaks, CA: Sage Publications, 1984.